EYES ON
JUNGLE DOCTOR

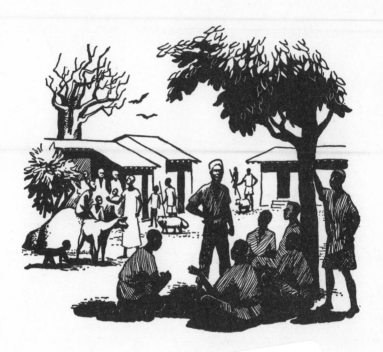

EYES ON
JUNGLE DOCTOR

Paul White

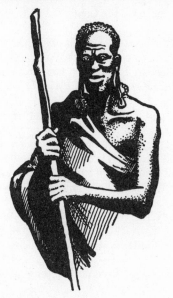

CF4·K

10 9 8 7 6 5 4 3 2

Eyes on Jungle Doctor ISBN 978-1-84550-393-2

© Copyright 1953 Paul White

First published 1953.

Reprinted 1954, 1956, 1958, 1961, 1963, 1965

Paperback edition 1972

by Paul White Productions,

4/1-5 Busaco Road, Marsfield, NSW 2122, Australia

Published in 2008 by Christian Focus Publications, Geanies House,
Fearn, Tain, Ross-shire, IV20 1TW, Scotland, U.K.

Reprinted in 2013

Fact files: © Copyright Christian Focus Publications

Cover design: Daniel van Straaten

Cover illustration: Craig Howarth

Interior illustrations: Helen M. Gillham

Printed and bound in Denmark by Nørhaven

*Since the Jungle Doctor books were first published there have been a
number of Jungle Doctors working in Mvumi Hospital, Tanzania, East
Africa - some Australian, some British, a West Indian and a number of
East African Jungle Doctors to name but a few.*

Scripture quotations taken from the HOLY BIBLE, NEW INTERNATIONAL
VERSION. Copyright © 1973, 1978, 1984 by International Bible Society.
Used by permission of Hodder & Stoughton Publishers.

Some Scripture quotations are based on the King James Version of the
Bible.

African words are used throughout the book, but explained at least once
within the text. A glossary is also included at the front of the book along
with a key character index.

CONTENTS

Fact File: Paul White

Born in 1910 in Bowral, New South Wales, Australia, Paul had Africa in his blood for as long as he could remember. His father captured his imagination with stories of his experiences in the Boer War which left an indelible impression. His father died of meningitis in army camp in 1915, and he was left an only child without his father at five years of age. He inherited his father's storytelling gift along with a mischievous sense of humour.

He committed his life to Christ as a sixteen-year-old schoolboy and studied medicine as the next step towards missionary work in Africa. Paul and his wife, Mary, left Sydney, with their small son, David, for Tanganyika in 1938. He always thought of this as his life's work but Mary's severe illness forced their early return to Sydney in 1941. Their daughter, Rosemary, was born while they were overseas.

Within weeks of landing in Sydney Paul was invited to begin a weekly radio broadcast which spread throughout Australia as the Jungle Doctor Broadcasts - the last of these was aired in 1985. The weekly scripts for these programmes became the raw material for the Jungle Doctor hospital stories - a series of twenty books.

Paul always said he preferred life to be a 'mixed grill' and so it was: writing, working as a Rheumatologist, public speaking, involvement with many Christian organisations, adapting the fable stories into multiple forms (comic books, audio cassettes, filmstrips), radio and television, and sharing his love of birds with others by producing birdsong cassettes - and much more.

The books in part or whole have been translated into 109 languages.

Paul saw that although his plan to work in Africa for life was turned on its head, in God's better planning he was able to reach more people by coming home than by staying. It was a great joy to meet people over the years who told him they were on their way overseas to work in mission because of the books.

Paul's wife, Mary, died after a long illness in 1970. He married Ruth and they had the joy of working together on many new projects. He died in 1992 but the stories and fables continue to attract an enthusiastic readership of all ages.

Fact File: Tanzania

The Jungle Doctor books are based on Paul White's missionary experiences in Tanzania. Today many countries in Africa have gained their independence. This has resulted in a series of name changes. Tanganyika is one such country that has now changed its name to Tanzania.

The name Tanganyika is no longer used formally for the territory. Instead the name Tanganyika is used almost exclusively to mean the lake.

During World War I, what was then Tanganyika came under British military rule. On December 9, 1961 it became independent. In 1964, it joined with the island of Zanzibar to form the United Republic of Tanganyika and Zanzibar, changed later in the year to the United Republic of Tanzania.

It is not only its name that has changed, this area of Africa has gone through many changes since the Jungle Doctor books were first written. Africa itself has changed. Many of the same diseases raise their heads, but treatments have advanced. However new diseases come to take their place and the work goes on.

Missions throughout Africa are often now run by African Christians and not solely by foreign nationals. There are still the same problems to overcome however. The message of the gospel thankfully never changes and brings hope to those who listen and obey. The Jungle Doctor books are about this work to bring health and wellbeing to Africa as well as the good news of Jesus Christ and salvation.

Fact File: Leprosy

Leprosy is one of the oldest recorded diseases. It is a chronic infectious disease that attacks the nervous system, particularly the nerves of the hands, feet and face. Sufferers feel no pain in these areas and are thus likely to injure themselves without realising it.

Leprosy is a painful condition which, although curable, can leave sufferers deformed and crippled if left untreated. It is caused by a bacteria similar to that which causes tuberculosis.

Lepromatous leprosy symptoms are a chronically stuffy nose and many skin lesions and nodules on the front and back of the body. Sensation loss starts at the fingers and toes and may only affect a small patch of skin to begin with. The loss of sensation can lead to unnoticed injuries which may in turn become infected. In advanced cases, gangrene will set in and flesh will rot on the patient.

Tuberculoid leprosy symptoms are a few well-defined skin lesions that are numb. Sensation loss may only affect a small patch of skin. Dimorphous leprosy creates skin lesions characteristic of the lepromatous and tuberculoid forms.

The disease is curable, but the effectiveness of the treatment is dependent on an early diagnosis.

Since 1982 the WHO has recommended multidrug therapy (MDT). Patients are given a cocktail of strong antibiotics which can completely cure the tuberculoid form of the disease within six months and the more infectious lepromatous form within two years.

Fact File: Meningitis

Meningitis is inflammation of the protective membranes covering the brain and spinal cord. It may develop most prominently in response to bacteria and viruses, but also physical injury, cancer or certain drugs. It is a serious condition. The most common form is treated with antibiotics and requires close observation. A severe headache is the most common symptom followed by neck stiffness.

Fact File: Words

WORDS TO ADD EXPRESSION AND EMPHASIS: Eh, Eeh, Hongo, Yah, Kah, Heh, Yah, Heheh Heeh, Ngh'eh, Huh, Heheeh, Hee, Yeh, Ooiyee, Weeh, Hodo, Koh, Hooh, Ukkkk, Heehee, Twi, Ooh, Ngheeh

TANZANIAN LANGUAGES: Swahili (main language), Chigogo or Gogo (one of the 150 tribal languages)

SENTENCES:

Alenyi wimbenyi - All together, sing

Alu Ng'hubita - I set out

Chai of saa kumi - Four in the afternoon

Chokwiwoni - We will see one another

Nhawule - What's up?

Nyamale - Be quiet

Yayagwe meso gakupaya paya - Oh my mother, my eyes they burn.

Zinghani na zinghani na zinghani - Words, words

WORDS IN ALPHABETICAL ORDER

Assante - Thank you

Bado - Not yet

Bwete - Hopeless

Chewi - Leopard

Cigongo - Back

Cipece - Cataract

Debe - Kerosene tin

Dudu - Insect

Fundi - Expert

Fundi kabisa - Great expert

Hodi - May I enter?

Ibalaluci - Thunder

Ibululu - Thornbush enclosure

Icewe - Jackal

Ichiligala - Eye ulcer

Icisi - The devil

Iganha - Egg

Igoda - Stool

Ikutupa - Tick

Ilwaliwa - Tortoise

Imuli -Lightning

Ituwi - Owl

Izuguni - Mosquito

Lunji - Perhaps

Karibu - Welcome

Kioo - Mirror

Kumbe - Behold!

Kwaheri - Goodbye

Macisi - The spirits

Madonga - Great store-bin

Malenga - Water

Mate - Spit

Mbeka - Truly

Mbisi - Hyena

Mbukwa - Good morning

Muganga - Witchdoctor

Mulungu - God, Supreme Being

Mutuka - Truck

Muzozi - Noisy one

Nhembo - Elephant

N'go - Never!

Nje - Scorpion

Pole - Gently

Saa kumi - Four in the afternoon

Sungura - Rabbit

Tabu sana - Great trouble

Ulange - Look

Upesi - Quickly

Wacho - Great One

Wiganga - Witchdoctors

Viswanu - All right

Winbe - Sing

Wuchawi - Witchcraft

Wugali - Porridge

Yayagwe - Oh my mother

Fact File: Characters

Berenge - Witchdoctor

Bibi - Grandmother, term of respect

Bwana - Dr White, main character/narrator

Cibofu - Blind man

Kefa - Nurse

Meshak - Patient

Mesomapya - Elderly chief

M'tendo - Sub chief

Naphthali - Previous patient

Ng'oma - Witchdoctor

Ng'ung'uliko - Grumbler

Ng'wagu - Old blind man

Petro - Head dispenser

Paolo - A blind teacher

Tadayo - Previous patient

Yacobo - Previous patient

Wazungu - Europeans

1
A Song and a Scorpion

I peered into the enormous mouth open in front of me. A large black finger pointed somewhat east of a not particularly entertaining looking tonsil, and a deep voice said:

'Bwana, it was there that great sorrow existed until the day when you with your weapons of iron caused it to cease.'

'*Hongo*,' said I politely, 'and how was it that this was attained, Tadayo?'

Nothing loth, the tall, very solid African in front of me went on with his story.

'*Yah*, Bwana, I came into the hospital over there.' He pointed with his chin, beyond an avenue of flame trees, to the C.M.S. Hospital. '*Yah*, Bwana, my hand was on my jaw, and behold it ached and ached. I came and I told you my story. You put me on a stool. You gave me medicine the colour of the sunset to wash my mouth with. I washed it for a long time, Bwana.'

How many times had I seen this thing! A dozen people armed with jam-tins full of purple solution, washing out their mouths, and ejecting with tremendous energy and surprising accuracy a squirt of purple fluid. Any black-beetle had a torrid time if it happened to come within range of my dental patients.

Tadayo was going on: '*Yah*, Bwana, and then you came with your tongs of iron and you said to me, "Open wide." Behold, I did, and you grasped my enemy firmly and fought with him. *Kah*, Bwana, how you fought! My hands firmly grasped the side of *igoda*, the stool. My neck was as strong as the trunk of a palm tree, and behold, Bwana, still you fought. *Hongo*, you fought with subtlety and strength. Did I not feel your wrist move this way and that way, but, behold, my enemy stuck to my jaw as *nhembo*, the elephant, stands with his feet firmly in a swamp. And, then Bwana, *heh*, when I thought all was lost, suddenly, *yah*, the victory was won! I saw him held in your tongs, Bwana, but sweat bathed my eyes, and the very tongs quivered in your hand because of your exertion.'

'*Hongo*,' said Daudi behind me, 'you're a man of many words. Did not the Bwana take his special forceps, and go "Hi!" and "Ho!" and there it was?'

'*Hongo*,' said Tadayo, 'do not the people say that I am the expert who tells the stories of the tribe, with great strength?'

'*Kumbe,* Bwana,' Daudi broke in, 'surely, Tadayo is indeed a *fundi*, an expert, when it comes to words.'

I looked at the smiling African before me. He was well into middle age. He seemed to ooze an air of cheerfulness. His eyes twinkled, but there was seriousness in his voice.

'Bwana, not only do I sing the songs of Tanganyika, but also I make up the songs of God. *Heh!* Many will listen to me sing, and behold, do I not suddenly bring in the songs of God, and they say "what words are these?" And then, behold, do I not tell them some stories from God's Book? Do I not tell them how Jesus came, how He lived? *Heh*, and they listen, for are not the words of God with great strength, and are they not as full of interest as is *iganha,* the egg, with food? Listen, Bwana, to our song.'

He turned to the people clustered round him. '*Alenyi wimbenyi* – all together, sing.'

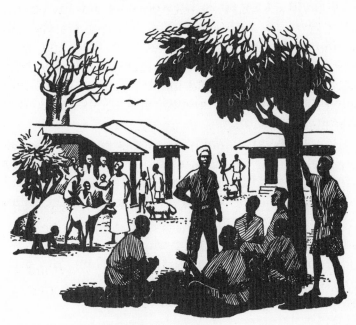

As they sang on, my eye took in the scene. The sky had a brazen look about it. The morning sun beat down upon the trees of the marketplace of this Central African town of Kilimatinde. In the background was the purple of bougainvillea creeping over the whitewashed walls, while the deep green of the mango trees showed near the market, where, beside a huge granite boulder, the usual bargaining was going on for beeswax, fat-tailed sheep, gaudy beads, kerosene and onions. A crow with beady eyes swung uncertainly on the bare branch of a flame tree, while a monkey on the broad limb of a baobab tree made an unhurried search in the hairs of its chest.

Suddenly, round the corner came an old man, dressed in a black cloth swung over his shoulder, and in his hand a long stick. He was being led by a small boy. Down the path they came towards us, the old man's feet feeling their way carefully before making each step. He came slowly up between the group of singers, stopped, groping with his hand, and then squatted down in the shade of the wall. The song came to an end.

'*Hongo,* Bwana,' said Tadayo, 'behold, one has come who is a master of singing. Is it not Ng'wagu who brings food to the ears of many at night round the fire? Behold, he knows all the songs of the tribe. *Heheh!* He sings them with energy.'

I put out my hand to the old man, who made no effort to shake it. I looked down at him. His eyes looked towards me, then vaguely his hand came out towards me. I gripped it in both of mine.

'*Mbukwa*, Ng'wagu, Good day,' I said, 'behold I have joy that you have visited us.'

My attention was riveted by his eyes. He had advanced cataract, the stark white centre of his eye speaking of eye lenses thickened, frosted and blocking out all but the full glare of the sun. Tadayo stood with his foot upon a large black stone on which he'd been sitting.

'Come,' he said, 'we sing again.'

The old man sang on. Tadayo came close to me, his amazingly large and flat toe pushing the stone upon which he had been sitting.

'Bwana,' he whispered, 'Ng'wagu is one to whom I have told the words of God. He has half understood them. Behold, this may be the other half.'

He stopped suddenly. His eyes rolled and he let out a roar, dragging his foot away from the stone, and at the same time bringing his knobbed stick down with a crash on the place where his toe had been, and I saw a scorpion in its death struggle. Tadayo was in acute pain. A scorpion bite is always agonising.

The singing broke up suddenly, and I said, 'Wait, I have medicine which will cure the pain.'

Tadayo followed me through the crowd of people, the small boys pressing behind to see what would happen. He sat on the step of the mission house while I anointed the spot with ointment, and then went inside to load a syringe of local anaesthetic. I was just sterilising a needle when a roar came from outside, and then the shrill danger signal. Daudi came running through the door.

'Bwana, great trouble! Great trouble! Your special medicine quickly!'

The alarm signal of the tribe rang out again. I picked up the sterilised syringe and a box of emergency injections and ran to the front steps of the mission house. People were standing there looking with horror at the broad form of Tadayo. He was leaning against the wall, fighting for breath, his lips an ugly blue colour and strangely swollen. A weird puffiness seemed to have come over one side of his face; his eye seemed to stick out.

'*Yayagwe, yayagwe,*' screamed an old African woman wringing her hands, 'this is the work of *wuchawi,* witchcraft!'

Some of the audience had taken to their heels. My hand was on Tadayo's pulse. I forced him into a sitting position and pushed his head down between his knees. I seized a small, sealed glass bottle from my medical emergency bag. Breaking the top off, I filled the syringe hurriedly and plunged the needle home into Tadayo's arm, injecting half the contents into his broad arm, and then turned to Daudi, saying in English:

'Get the largest spoon you can find and be very quick.'

He rushed off. I spoke quietly to Tadayo.

'This is a bad thing. It is because of the bite that you have received from *Nje,* the scorpion. Behold, we call this *allergy.* Is there not a swelling across the place where you make your words, and in the large path that the breath comes to and from your lungs? The medicine that I am giving you will overcome this trouble. Do not struggle. If your wisdom seems small and your head reels, still keep quiet, keep calm. Soon I will put the wrong end of a large spoon into your mouth. We will open the way for air to go in. Have small fear. Have we not the medicines of great strength? They will bring safety and security and they will keep life within your body.'

Daudi was at my side with a spoon. 'Take the syringe,' I ordered, 'and inject one drop every minute. Count sixty slowly. When you reach that number, inject.'

The African dispenser nodded.

I bent down and sitting on one of the steps, was able to force Tadayo's teeth apart and to push his tongue back. There was a little gulp of air. I spoke on reassuringly.

'All is well. We are overcoming it. Behold, before long, *heh,* all will be itself again. It is like the thunderstorm rushing across the sky, making such a noise.'

I saw Daudi's finger move on the plunger. A shudder went through Tadayo's body. The swelling round his lips became less. His great hand was on my bare knee. He squeezed.

'*Heh,*' I said, 'it's coming right.'

Beneath me, old Ng'wagu the African singer was standing, his head at an unusual angle. His eyes being out of commission, his ears were playing almost a double role. He was tense, taking in every happening.

Again Daudi's fingers moved. Tadayo's eye seemed to have gone back more into position. He put his hand on my arm, trying to tell me that he wanted the spoon removed from his mouth.

I did so.

His lips were moving, and I caught the word.

'*Malenga*, water.'

I motioned for this to be brought. Again Daudi moved his finger on the plunger.

'Bwana, that is all the injections.'

'Right. Out with the needle. Rub the spot; rub it hard.' Daudi did so.

The water was brought. Tadayo drank and then drew in air with a long, hesitant breath.

'*Hongo*,' he gasped, 'Bwana, *heh*, I thought I had passed through the gates of death.'

'Truly, my friend, you came close to them, but fortunately I was here, and I had the medicine. *Hongo*, keep away from scorpions! That *dudu* has not only a poison in his tail which brings pain, but he's got a very special poison that does very strange things to you.'

I took the cotton wool from Daudi's hand and rubbed vigorously where the injection had been given, and then speaking in a tone that only my patient could hear, I said:

'Perhaps within your life, Tadayo, there is a special sin, a pet, favourite sin, and may not this very amazing happening be a warning to you from God?'

The tall African turned to me. 'Bwana, how did you know?' And then he realised what he had said. He looked down at the ground. 'Bwana,' he said, 'your words are words of truth. Behold this *is* a warning. I have preached many words but inside me was evil.' He shook his head.

Ng'wagu's deep voice came from just behind us.

'Bwana,' he said, 'tell me. What is happening? What has happened? Tell me it all; I want to know.'

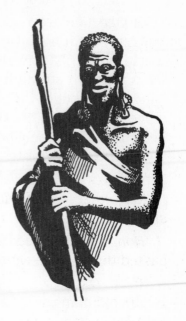

I took him by the arm, noticing that his ear lobe was vastly pierced and full of all sorts of ornaments, mainly beadwork, threaded on giraffe hairs. Ornaments made from solder and ornaments cut from native wood were there. His hair was in tight curls, some of them grey, some of them black. There was a long scar over his shoulder, a knife wound. I placed my hand near this scar.

'Great One, behold, this is the word of strange sickness. Tadayo had his foot beside a flat stone. He pushed it with his toe. *Nje*, the scorpion, was beneath that stone. It objected to Tadayo's disturbing it, and behold, it bit his toe.'

'*Hongo!*' Ng'wagu nodded vigorously.

'And, behold, the bite of *Nje*, the scorpion, is full of pain.'

'*Eh, eh*,' said Tadayo, 'those words are true. But behold, the Bwana had medicine to put on it which quickly stopped the pain; it was medicine of strength.'

'Truly,' I said, 'but the poison of *Nje* not only produced pain at the place where it bit you, but did it not upset all of you?'

21

'*Hongo*,' Tadayo nodded vigorously, 'it was weird. Suddenly my tongue swelled, my lips swelled, my eye would not go back within the cover of its lid, and I felt as though strong hands were pressing upon my windpipe. I fought for breath. I thought death would come. But, behold, Bwana, you came and pushed my head down, and then, *heh*, the bite of the needle, and you talked quiet words.'

'*Hongo*,' said Ng'wagu, 'I heard all of this, but I did not see. Many will think it is the work of evil spirits.'

'*Heh*,' I said, 'or perhaps a very strong spell, eh? It isn't though. We have a strong medicine that cures it.'

The old man's hand came round. He looked at me with his unseeing eyes.

'Bwana,' he said, 'have you other strong medicines for bad diseases?'

'It is even so.'

'Bwana, behold, I walk in darkness. I cannot see. Is... is... there... anything...?'

'*Heeh*, we can help you. There are many others who have suffered as you suffer, and they have been helped. But sit down upon the steps here. Behold, we will drink tea and talk of these things.'

'*Heeh*,' grunted Tadayo, 'I could drink tea.'

The people were slowly coming round us again. My tea and Tadayo's came in cups, but they had put Ng'wagu's in a gourd. The old man put it to his lips and drank with a sucking noise. I smiled and turned to the people.

'Behold, is there any fear in the disease which may be conquered by a medicine which is still stronger?'

'Bwana,' they said, 'there is no fear in this.'

Tadayo was seated just behind me.

'Bwana, behold, there is one here upon whose eye you operated, as you will work on the eye of Ng'wagu, if he will permit you. Behold, he has words.'

The old blind man sat hunched up, scratching the sole of his foot.

'Great One,' I said, 'behold, there is one here who will bring joy to your ears. This is Naphthali.'

Ng'wagu sat upright. '*Nhawule,* how can this be?'

'What are your words, Naphthali?'

The African leant forward. 'Behold, Bwana, in the days when you first came here was I not one of the blind? Did I not walk in darkness? But, behold, things are different now, since you worked on my eye with your instruments.'

Ng'wagu was on his feet. He stumbled forward. 'I would know the truth of these words,' he said. 'I would know them.'

2
Utitu - The Land of Darkness

Naphthali held up his hand for silence.

'Behold, when I walked, if there was a hole anywhere near, *heh*, would I not fall into it?' he held up his foot for our inspection. 'Do you not see the burns? Have I not walked into the fire, and the hot ashes? *Yah*, how they gave pain! But, *hongo*, how shall one who lives in the land of Utitu, in darkness, know when his foot is going into a hole or into the fire?'

Ng'wagu nodded his head vigorously.

'*Heh*, how well I know these things. Behold, do not your feet acquire great skill to tell you where you are going when you are on a path? Can you not feel the sides of it? But, behold, in other places, how are you to know?'

'*Heh*,' nodded Naphthali, 'these are words of truth. Behold, many is the bruise, many is the scar that I gained through walking in darkness, and then came one who said to me:

"Behold, at Mvumi, way out across the plain, there is *Mzungu*, a European, who has great skill to deal with people's eyes."'

I looked across at Daudi and winked. He smiled back, for both of us knew just how difficult things had been in the early days, when I had not done much surgical work as far as eyes were concerned, and when my hand wobbled in such a way as to destroy the confidence of anyone but a blind man. My mind went back still further to the days, shortly after my graduation, when with two medical degrees and very little experience I had operated on scores of pigs' eyes set in plasticine, doing the tricky procedure of lens extraction, the basis of the cataract operation.

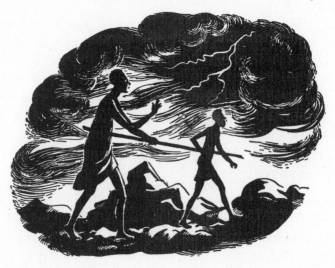

The old African's voice went on. 'I called one of my family, a small boy, and we walked. *Heh*, it was a great safari. It was the days of the rains, and *imuli*, the lightning, flashed through the sky. I knew it, for suddenly I would see just a hint of light, and then *ibalaluci* – the thunder – roared in its anger, and we stood under trees while the rivers from the hills pelted down. We heard the voices of the animals at night and had fear. But, Bwana, I sought for light, and always I thought "at the end of this safari is the thing that will help me." And then we came to Mvumi. *Heheh*, how I remember it. You looked at my eyes. You pulled the lids up. You turned me to the sun and said, "Can you see anything?" And I said, "*Heeh*, I see redness." And you said, "Good." And then you turned to me again, and you said,"Do you see anything?" And I said, "No, blackness only!"'

'*Heh*,' said Daudi, 'Bwana, you said to me, "His retina is all right."'

The old man who had cataracts now and was in darkness put his head up. 'Retina?' he said, 'retina? A word I know not.'

'It is at the back of the eye,' I said. 'It catches the light as *kioo*, the mirror, collects a picture upon its surface.'

'*Kumbe*,' said the old man, nodding slowly. 'What happened after the Bwana examined your eye?'

Naphthali went on with his story. 'They put me to bed and kept me there many days. They taught me many things; to obey, not to be frightened. They washed my face very frequently. They put much medicine into my eyes. I drank much medicine. They massaged my back with medicine that smelt.'

Daudi looked at me and grinned. His lips framed the words, 'methylated spirits.'

'And then the day came when the Bwana took me to the place that he called "operating theatre." *Yah*, but so great was my excitement that I forget. I forget what happened there. *Hongo*, but I will never forget what happened when the Bwana took off my bandage. I saw. I *saw! Hongo*, and I still see!'

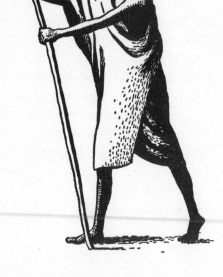

Ng'wagu was on his feet. He came across to me – surely, purposefully, his hands outstretched.

'Bwana, that I too might receive my sight.'

I took his two hands in mine and said, 'Listen, Great One, I would tell you of one who made just such a request of One whom I call my Lord. It was this way.

'Jesus was on safari, going to a town called Jericho. Beside the road sat a blind man, asking people for food, for money. He heard a lot of people going by. He asked them, "What's it all about?" Many passed, but one stopped and said, "*Hongo*, do you not know? Jesus of Nazareth is passing by. He's on safari."'

'The blind man stood to his feet and shouted, "Jesus, Son of David, take pity on me."

'Those that passed said, "*Nyamale* – be quiet." But the more they said it, the louder he shouted. "Oh, Son of David, take pity on me."

'And Jesus stopped and said, "Bring him to me." As he came close Jesus asked him, "What do you want me to do for you?"

'He said, "Bwana, let me get back my sight." And as he stood there before Jesus there was silence, and then Jesus said, "Regain your sight. It is your faith that has done this."

'*Hongo*, they were amazed, for instantly the man got his sight back and he followed Jesus, praising God with many words.'

Old Ng'wagu swung round, 'Faith,' he said, 'what is that? Make it so that I can understand.'

Daudi had an answer. 'Naphthali had faith. He heard what the Bwana could do. He walked to the hospital because he thought the Bwana could do it. He let the Bwana work on his eye. He heard; he went; he obeyed. The Bwana worked on his eye and, behold, he saw. Faith is trusting and letting what you trust in happen.'

'*Hongo*,' said the old man slowly.

Tadayo could sense that the old man didn't know what to do, so eased the tension by breaking into one of his songs. The others, including Ng'wagu, joined in the chorus.

I saw Daudi work his way through the group standing near and run across towards the marketplace. I wondered what it was all about. And then I saw him take a small boy by the arm and lead him slowly towards me. The singers went on enthusiastically.

Daudi's voice came clearly to me, 'Bwana, here is a child with very bad eyes. Behold, how bad they are.'

The boy was about eleven. His eyes were red and raw-looking, his face streaked with tears and discharge. He held his hand over his eyes and screwed them up because of the glare of the midday sun.

I whispered to Daudi, 'Get hold of the microscope. Bring it round here.' Then I spoke aloud. 'Behold,' I said, 'see the child's eyes. Are they eyes of joy?'

There was a shaking of heads. They knew only too well what would happen to this child if he were given the medicines of the *waganga*, the witchdoctors. Here was another recruit for the great army of the blind in Tanganyika. But I knew that inside, in the kerosene-driven refrigerator, which was the latest weapon in our hospital, were penicillin drops which in a matter of twenty-four hours would change the whole situation.

Daudi had come back with the microscope. With a sterilised glass rod I took a little of the material from the corner of the lad's eye, and put it on a slide. Daudi focused the microscope out there in the sunlight. *'Ulange*, Bwana, look,' he said, pointing to the eyepiece. There was the germ that was causing the trouble.

I tried to show it to them but no one would look into the microscope except Tadayo, and he smiled.

'Yah,' he said, 'it looks like two little beans with a fence around them.' He proceeded to model in the sand what he saw.

I said, *'Heh*, and we have the medicine that can cure this.'

To the child I said, 'Stay here with us for some days. Daudi will put drops into your eyes. There will be no pain. Behold, before the setting of the sun you will see whether this medicine works.'

The drops were put in and the boy was given an eye-shade made from the cover of the *East African Standard*. Old Ng'wagu had run his fingertips over the small boy's face.

'*Yah*,' he said, 'I know this trouble. It is a very bad one indeed, Bwana. Many children are blinded because of it.'

'Great One,' I said, 'tonight as the sun sets we will once again bring the child to you. And behold, his eyes will have much less trouble and in three days he will have eyes as normal as those of his companions.'

'*Hongo*,' replied the old man, 'this is a thing of wonder, Bwana.'

Then he tapped me on the arm. 'This Jesus that you told me about, can he do now what He did then?'

'Yes,' I said, 'but He is not with us in the way that we can see. He died.'

'*Yah*,' said the old minstrel, 'before He could help me.'

'But listen, He is no longer dead. Behold, he sends people to do His work. I am one of them.'

'*Kah*,' said Ng'wagu, 'how can all this be?'

'Stay with us,' I replied, 'we will show you.'

3

Dark Safari

The small African boy with two horribly inflamed eyes sat in the shade on the back porch of the Mission House. The sun was directly overhead. It was midday, time to put more drops into his eyes. I took them out of the refrigerator, loaded the dropper, told him to open his eyes wide and in went the drops.

'Bwana,' he said, 'they do not hurt, not even a little bit!'

'*Ngh'eh*,' I nodded, 'they do not hurt you, but the *dudus*, the little germs in your eyes, *heh*, they have no joy in that medicine. It is strong poison for them.'

The small boy laughed gleefully. '*Heh*, Bwana, sorrow to them is joy to me.'

Again I nodded. 'Come again, when the sun has reached this point.'

I held my hand to show where the sun would be at four o'clock. Daudi took hold of the metal tray, with its array of medicines, swabs and droppers.

'*Yah*, Bwana!' He shook his hands as though they were burning. 'Never have I touched anything as cold as that! Truly, this is a cupboard of great wisdom. Where did it come from?'

'One of my friends gave me this. It was sent out here so that we might keep the medicines that have great strength. This penicillin, *heh*, it will save many eyes, and behold, the babies' milk.' I pointed to a number of big bottles, full to the brim. 'We can keep that for many days. Germs cannot breed fast when they are in the cold. Very many things can be done with one of these. It is a real weapon to help us.'

'*Heh*,' said Daudi, 'and over there in the corner, Bwana. Are we not keeping the various test-tubes that we use in our pathology?'

'Truly, Daudi, never was a hundred pounds spent better than on this machine.'

Four o'clock came and with it the small boy. His eyes were looking better already, but more drops went in. At five o'clock there was quite a commotion outside. I saw old Ng'wagu, the blind man, coming along. With him were two folk with a strange African instrument made from umbrella spokes flattened and mounted on what looked like a cigar box. They were twanging away, and chanting softly. It seemed we were in for a musical evening.

Soon a crowd of Africans had gathered and they swayed to the playing of the musician.

Ng'wagu spoke. 'Behold, that is the playing of a *fundi* – an expert.'

'*Heh*, Great One,' I said, 'truly, but behold, I would hear your voice. Sing to us the song of the girls who were lost in the mountains as they were cutting firewood.'

The old man tossed his head back and sung huskily.

Song followed song, and then sunset came…a gorgeous sunset. I stood there watching it, the music throbbing on behind me, and the African voices forming their own strange background. Darkness was falling, then came a small voice behind me.

'Bwana, I have come for medicine.'

It was the small boy who at noon had two extremely bad eyes … here he was with eyes that looked almost normal. There was a little redness but the swelling had gone, and the discharge, too. Penicillin certainly works at an amazing rate. I duly put in drops again, and then took him down to where the folk were all gathered singing. I held up my hand for silence.

'Look, Great Ones, here is the child who was with us this morning. See how he is now.'

Tadayo stood up and looked at the child. The sky above us was brilliantly red. He looked at the child's eyes. They were white. He looked at the sky again. 'O Great One, behold, in a matter of hours the child's eyes have changed from the colour of the sky to the colour of milk.'

Ng'wagu struggled to his feet and groped his way forward. He put his hands over the child's face, his fingers moving over the closed eyelids.

'*Hongo*,' he said, 'to me this seems a thing of wonder.'

The child spoke up. '*Heh*, it *is* a thing of wonder. The pain has gone, the soreness also.'

'Behold,' I said, 'O Great Ones, remember that we have very strong medicine for eyes. Do we not follow out the words of our Bwana, Jesus? Did He not say, "I am the Light of the world"? Is it therefore not a good thing to bring back light to ordinary eyes, that people may see with the eyes of their soul?'

They all got up and said *kwaheri* – goodbye. I watched Tadayo and Ng'wagu in earnest discussion.

The sun had set, the reds went to purple, the purple to deep blue. The stars came out surprisingly quickly. Darkness had come, darkness that restricted your movements, darkness you could almost feel. I turned to go across to the door and nearly fell, stumbling over Ng'wagu's walking-stick. Away in the hills I could hear the drums and the singing of Africans.

Two dark figures loomed up before me. Their silhouettes made it obvious that they were Tadayo and Ng'wagu.

Tadayo whispered into my ear. 'Ng'wagu would have special words with you.'

'Bwana,' said the old man, 'may I come with you on safari to Mvumi? I, too, would like you to work upon my eyes that I might see.'

'*Heeh*, Ng'wagu, I will have joy to try and help you. We continue our safari tomorrow, travelling from place to place. Perhaps we shall have opportunity to take you part of the way in the truck, but you will have to journey many miles on foot.

'*Heh*, Bwana, I would have joy to do this.'

'Perhaps the safari will have danger in it and difficulty.'

The old blind man shrugged his shoulders. 'Will it not be worth while if light returns?'

It was an eerie night. *Ituwe*, the owl, sat far out on the limb of a great baobab tree. Bats fluttered around in the starlight. Berenge, the witchdoctor, whose great medicine was for eyes, rocked to and fro on his three-legged stool, looking at the moon silhouetted roundly against the deep blue of the night sky. He thought of the grain in his *madonga,* the great store-bin, and of his sheep and cattle and goats in the *ibululu*, the thornbush enclosure, which kept away leopards and lions and hyenas and jackals.

To his ear, on the warm breeze of the night, came the singing of the Wagogo, the people of Central Tanganyika. They sang in the village and played their games. Berenge had contentment, for had he not that day added a kerosene tin full of millet to his store, and a large white goat to his flock? Had he not made medicine for the child of M'tendo? But his contentment lasted for a short time only. Suddenly a scowl came over his face and he spat into the dying fire, for away on the hill, beyond the spring, where the women draw water, a strong light moved and swung out over the plain. Again Berenge spat and reached for his drum.

* * *

Up on the hill, an old truck pulled up in front of the Makutapora leprosy settlement. Both doors swung open and a voice said:

'Open up the back and let the old man out, Daudi. He'll be stiff after that drive.'

The hurricane-lantern was lighted and the back of the car opened. An old African, dusty and very tired-looking, struggled to his feet. His eyes stared, unblinking and unseeing, at the light of the lamp. His

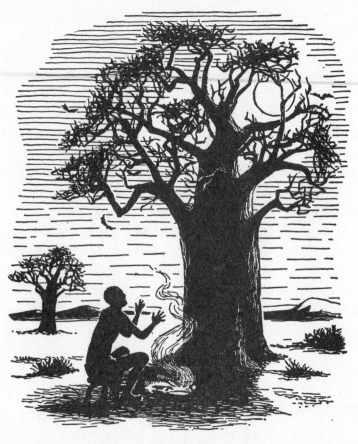

legs were gingerly stretched over the back of the car. He touched the ground.

'*Yoh,* my legs are stiff with much sitting. *Kumbe*, and my tongue … *heh* … it is dry with much dust. Does not the *mutuka*, the truck, move with the motion of a giraffe? *Kumbe,* and does it not bring strife to those who ride in it? *Kah*, Bwana, I would taste water.'

A moment or two later, Daudi came up with a three-legged stool and a gourd of water. Ng'wagu drank deeply and with great satisfaction.

'*Yah,*' he said, sitting on the stool, 'but I have a famine within me.'

'*Heh,* food will follow, but first let me put drops into your eyes, so that there may be no germs, that the dust may not cause them any trouble which would stop the Bwana from operating.'

The old man tilted his head back and the African adroitly put drops into each eye, and a faint smudge of ointment across the eyelids. For a moment there was silence and then came the distant throb of a drum. The old man stirred uneasily.

'*Kumbe,*' he muttered, 'that is the voice of the drum of Berenge, the witchdoctor. I know him. His medicines are strong.'

Further down the hill in a darker shadow in the darkness of the night was another house – mud walls, mud roof, mud floors – built U-shaped with square corners, the open end being blocked with thornbush. Within this the cattle stamped, and the goats moved quietly, stirring restlessly as they heard the voice of *icewe*, the jackal. Inside on a cowskin tossed a boy, the eldest son of M'tendo, the sub-chief. He groaned and then suddenly he cried:

'Oh, my mother – *yayagwe meso gakupaya paya* – my eyes, they burn, they burn.'

'*Nyamale,* be quiet,' came the voice of M'tendo, but the child continued to whimper.

'*Heh*, my eyes, they burn, how they burn, how they burn.'

'*Hongo,*' said an old man sitting before the fire, 'behold, has not the child had the medicine of Berenge, and is not Berenge one of wisdom in the medicines for eyes?'

From somewhere within the mud house came the pathetic, insistent crying of the child, '*Yah*, my eyes, how they burn, my eyes, my eyes.'

Clearly, almost ominously, on the night air came the sound of the drums. The old man sitting before the fire said, 'Behold, there is no peace in the heart of Berenge, the witchdoctor, this night. Is it that he has no joy in the medicines that he has made?'

'*Kah,*' said M'tendo, 'this cannot be. Berenge is *fundi kabisa*, a great expert.'

'*Heh,*' said the old man querulously, 'but the child of Madila. Behold, did not Berenge make medicines for his eyes and, *heh*, behold, he is no more. Is this the work of an expert?'

'*Kah*,' said M'tendo, 'those are words of no purpose.'

The drum of Berenge came more loudly on the night air.

'*Heh,*' said the old man getting up from his seat beside the fire and shuffling inside the house, 'behold, Berenge walks this night.'

M'tendo stood beside the dying embers of the fire listening as the sound of the drum came up and up in volume. Then he seemed to hear it calling to him. He picked up his stick and walked off into the darkness, hardly noticing the thornbush that reached out to drag at his cloth as he walked down the narrow path. Dimly he heard the noise made by the baboons on the hillside as they whimpered in terror, knowing that that night *chewi,* the leopard, was hunting. He had ears only for the drum of Berenge. The broken rhythm changed to an insistent beat, and suddenly stopped. M'tendo found himself underneath a great baobab tree, standing face to face with the witchdoctor, whose eyes seemed to shine out of the gloom at him.

'*Hongo,*' said Berenge, 'I have the words of *Icisi,* the devil, who is my particular servant. He tells me that Wazungu, the Europeans, from the hospital at Mvumi are coming this way, and I warn you that should they give medicine to your child he will die, and die quickly.'

'*Hongo,*' muttered M'tendo, 'Great One, I will follow your wisdom.'

Berenge spat, and lifted his hands on high with his drum in them. 'Woe will come to our village if these people come.'

Overhead at that moment flew *ituwi,* the owl, perching on a branch just above our heads.

'Behold,' said Berenge, pointing upwards with his chin, '*Icisi,* the devil, sends his messenger that my warning may have greater strength.'

He took up his drum and beat softly.

Back in the house of M'tendo, the child rolled in agony on his couch, and suddenly the whole of his body was shaken with shivers. His teeth chattered and he cried out, 'My father, I have great cold in my body, but my eyes burn and burn.'

'*Nyamale*, be quiet,' whispered the old man from further inside the hut, but the child continued to shiver in spasms, his teeth chattering convulsively together like the rattles of the dancers at the tribal initiations, and then the spasm passed off, and the child, almost in a whisper said:

'O Lord God, You of whom they speak and sing at the hospital on the hill, O God, bring me help.'

He raised his voice, repeating the words again. His eyes were sightless or he would have seen, framed in the doorway, his father, his face contorted with anger.

He came across to the child, kicked him with his foot, dragged the cowskin from under him and left him lying naked on the floor. Through the stillness of the night came the drum of Berenge, rising and falling on the night air.

On the hill Daudi stood listening.

'*Kah*, Bwana, that drum is an evil drum. It brings a message of fear to the heart of old Ng'wagu. He knows what it says. He is of the old ones of the tribe, and they understand better than I do. But, behold, Bwana, there is witchcraft in the air; there is devilry. This is what we call the black wisdom.' The African shivered.

'*Hongo*, Daudi, I can feel it in my bones too, but do you remember in God's Book how Daniel was in great trouble? Everyone said he would be killed. Was he not thrown into a cave containing lions, unfed to make them fierce? But the jealous ones who did this to him did not know that God Himself was there to protect, to help. Did He not shut the mouths of the lions? It was a thing of wonder, but remember, the God who helped him will help us. He is just the same God. Behold, we will see His power to help us before this night is out.'

Behind me came the voice of Petro, the African head dispenser of the leprosy settlement.

'Here's work, Bwana, dangerous work. Over in the village of Sasagila, one of my black-sheep families; *huh*, they're a trial; they will not take their medicines; they wear charms where injections are needed; they kill a goat and make offering to the ancestors when they need the help of the hospital. Always it is the word of Berenge, the witchdoctor, that they follow. They have seen that our medicines work better, but, behold, they still turn to the old ways.'

'How did you hear about this, Petro?'

'I have this word from an old man whose ulcer we cured.'

'*Hongo*,' I raised my eyebrows, 'tell me, what mistakes of the witchdoctor do we have to clear up now?'

'A small boy called M'dogo, behold, he has the disease.' He pointed his chin towards the leprosy hospital. Daudi and I nodded. 'His eyes have been in trouble. He was taken to the witchdoctor, who has made his usual medicine by chewing up leaves and cactus juice and spitting them into the eye of the child. Behold, Bwana, his disease has made him very ill. They say his eyes are destroyed and that his body burns like fire.'

Daudi was already going over the stocks of medicines.

'*Kah*,' he said, 'this will require penicillin. There is small doubt that the child has blood-poisoning. This is a thing we have seen so very, very often. *Heh*, will the Waganga never follow the ways of wisdom? Behold their eye medicine. *Kah!*' Daudi spat with deep disgust into the darkness.

I have seldom had a journey in which there were silhouettes more eerie than the limbs of thornbush and of baobab trees, like bony arms of a skeleton, standing out gaunt against the deep blue of the night sky.

'There's a peculiar stillness about the night, Daudi.'

'*Heheeh*, Bwana, when *chewi*, the leopard, is stalking baboons they are quiet. *Chewi* himself makes no noise.'

There came a throbbing of drums from down in the plain: a slow tempo, an ominous noise. We came to the huts. The drum seemed to throb more loudly as we came to the door we sought. No one answered our '*Hodi.*' We pushed the wicker door open to be assailed by an odour of stale wood smoke and goats. The smoky hurricane-lantern opened up a picture of Central African life which sent a shudder down my spine. The small boy lay naked on the bare ground, his eyes sightless, unbelievably swollen, and showing starkly the dreadful effects of the witchdoctor's work.

We wrapped him in a blanket and made him as comfortable as we could. My finger on his pulse was barely able to detect the fluttering of his heart. I slipped a thermometer under his arm and to my amazement I found that the mercury reached almost the limit. He was 109°. I looked up at the faces standing out oddly in the yellow light of the hurricane-lamp. Daudi just nodded his head. He realised that the child was beyond medical aid. The child's lips moved. I could hear no sound, but Daudi understood. He bent down, lifted the little chap's head, and gave him a drink of water from the gourd. His lips were moving again.

'Bwana, I asked God that you might come. *Winbe* – sing,' he whispered.

Very softly Petro sang:

> There is a city bright,
> Closed are its gates to sin,
> Nothing that's tainted
> Can ever enter in.

The small boy lifted himself on his elbow. 'Bwana, but has God not taken away my sin, my taint?'

I bent down close to him. 'You asked Him to, did you not?'

'*Heh*, Bwana, I did.'

'Did the Son of God lie?'

'*Kumbe* – no,' said the small boy. 'He would not lie.'

'Therefore the gates are open to you.'

'*Heh*, Bwana, *heh*, the gates are open to me.' He sank back smiling.

Beyond the lamplight I was conscious of figures moving. A cockroach scuttled across the floor, and outside the drums throbbed.

My fingers were on the small boy's pulse. The fluttering for a moment was accentuated and then stopped. Petro was holding the other wrist.

'Bwana, he has already passed through those gates.'

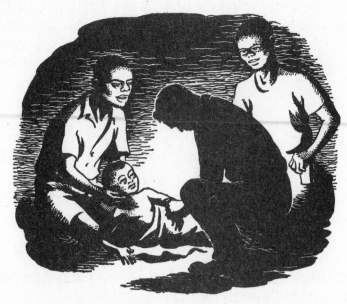

I looked round at the squalor of that mud hut, the filth, the patch of active leprosy on the small boy's face. Daudi watched my eyes, and said in a voice barely above a whisper, 'Bwana, surely the reason is clear why we have our hospital up there, for ones like this.'

Suddenly we were aware of a crowd of people at the door. There was a harsh voice: 'Your medicines have failed. You have damaged the child.'

'*Kumbe,*' said Petro, 'behold, our medicines have not even been given; the work of Berenge, the witchdoctor, has produced the death of the child.'

When they heard that the child was dead, the women started to give the death howl, and an old man blew on a cow's horn the distress signals of the tribe.

Daudi whispered, 'Bwana, we'd better get out of this. There's nothing we can do. They will not listen to us. They will work themselves up into a frenzy. It were better that we left.'

Petro nodded. '*Heh*, Bwana, these are words of wisdom.'

We moved out into the pallor of the moonlight. In front of us stood M'tendo, the child's father.

'*Kah,*' he said, 'from the hospital you produce medicines. You say these medicines work. They did not cure the child.'

'*Heh,*' said Petro, 'does a man grow in strength if he eats food but once a week? Shall people recover from this disease if they do not take the medicines in the way in which they are told?'

'*Kah,*' said M'tendo, ignoring Petro. 'You talk many words. You say that leprosy is like sin. I' – he smacked himself loudly on the chest – 'I have sinned?'

'*Hongo,*' said Daudi, 'the Words of God are these. "If we say that we have no sin, we deceive ourselves," and nobody else. Truly we deceive not God, nor men.'

'*Yah,*' said M'tendo. His long-knobbed stick swung through the air viciously.

He drew closer till suddenly Berenge moved out of the darkness. His eyes were piercing. He fixed them on me and slowly drew a circle on the ground with his foot on a place where my footprints stood out clearly

Then slowly he turned, the leopard's teeth on his neck swayed and the white ivory witchdoctors' ornaments showed up as he stalked off into the darkness.

'*Yoh,*' said Daudi, 'a spell against you, Bwana, of very great strength.'

M'tendo was cowering back obviously terrified.

I turned to Daudi and Petro. 'Come on. Let's get back; we must do two things: first help Ng'wagu, and then be ready for any tricks Berenge may see fit to play.'

Petro looked grim. 'Bwana, make no mistake. He will attack us before the night is old.'

'*Hee!*' grinned Daudi. 'The Bwana has a trick that will surprise Berenge. Surely it is a trap of subtlety.'

4
Trap for Witchdoctors

'If you want to catch a witchdoctor, Petro, the thing to do is to set a trap. First you need a *debe,* a kerosene tin, and a lot of string. Fix the string loosely across the path about three inches above the ground, and, behold, your witchdoctor's feet pull the string and the tin goes "crash" in the way that *debes* do.'

'That's a good idea, Bwana, especially when there are few paths and much thornbush. Will we not then stretch string across the path so that should Beregne come to cast spells and walk around the house in the way that witchdoctors do, then behold, he will find something that will give him fear in his heart?'

'*Hongo,*' said Daudi, behind me, 'Bwana, it is well you spoke those words in English. If Ng'wagu had heard that, he would have great fear within himself. Did not Berenge say that he changes himself into the shape of *mbisi,* the hyena?'

'*Kumbe*, Daudi, that is no new thing. We have a witchdoctor near Mvumi who changes himself into a lion! Behold, Berenge must be only a second-class witchdoctor to change himself into a dead-meat-eating hyena.'

Daudi grinned. 'Bwana, there are more hyenas in this part of Tanganyika than there are lions, so, behold, it is a good thing to change yourself into a hyena. Behold, is not the voice of *mbisi* and his many relations lifted up each night? The people say Berenge is hunting; Berenge is casting spells. *Kah*, it is a good thing that he makes strong medicines on our behalf. Behold, the spell will not be cast on me. So Berenge grows rich and grows fat, and sits beside his fire. *Mbisi*, the hyena, earns him money.'

'Right, come on. Let's set our traps. You get the tins, Daudi. I'll get the string.'

Five minutes later we started to prepare things.

'*Kah*, Bwana, there are not many *debes* round this place, but I found other tins as well. I found this near the kitchen. It has a little bit of cooking-fat in the bottom, Bwana. *Kah,* it smells!' Daudi wrinkled his nose.

'*Hongo*, that won't upset the noise that the tin makes! We'll use it. Tie the string on to that hole in the side. *Yeh,* that's the idea.'

In the moonlight nine traps were set. The string was hardly visible to anyone who was not looking for it. Every path to the hospital was covered. In some cases there were two traps.

I went up to the room where the old man was sitting, huddled up on the floor, shivering.

'Ng'wagu,' I said, 'you have no joy.'

'*Eeh*, Bwana, there is fear in my heart. Berenge casts spells. He would keep me in darkness and, Bwana, his medicines are strong ones. Behold, I have fear. All thoughts of mine have gone from my head. I hear only the sound of the drum of Berenge. Bwana, it says words that bring fear to me. It says, "the Bwana is overcome by the wisdom of Berenge."'

Ng'wagu rocked to and fro. *'Ooiyee!'* he crooned in despair. 'Berenge is a witchdoctor of great strength and is not *mbisi*, the hyena, his helper? Truly the strenth of *mbisi* is great. I can feel it, Bwana. I can feel it with strength.'

'*Hongo*, is Berenge greater than *Mulungu*, God, who created him?'

'*Weeh*,' said the old man. 'Behold, Bwana, Berenge has the strength of the devil. *Macisi,* the spirits, are his servants. *Hongo*, and *mbisi,* the hyena, is his messenger. Listen…'

In the distance, on the night air, came the cry of a hyena.

'*Hongo*,' I said disgustedly. 'I'll teach Berenge about hyenas.'

But little did I guess…

I turned down the hurricane-lantern to a mere glimmer and opened the door, looking out over the plains that lay still before us in dull, metallic colour.

In an excited whisper Daudi reported, 'Bwana, the tins are tied. Every path has its trap.'

We stood looking out over the still greyness. Ng'wagu from the background said in a husky voice,

'Daudi, tell me of the things that you see, that within my head I may understand, although my eyes are shut to the things of the night.'

'*Kah*,' said Daudi beside me, 'that is a fine mixture of words, Bwana.'

I grinned and then, closer at hand, came the weird laughter of *mbisi*. Ng'wagu struggled to his feet, knocking over his little stool.

'*Kah*,' he said, 'it is Berenge himself. He has taken upon him the body of *mbisi*. He is coming. Within me I know it. He will cast a spell against me so that darkness will remain in my eyes. *Kah*, I have fear! I have fear!' His voice reached an hysterical pitch.

Daudi was beside the old man, sitting him down again on his stool, and speaking soothingly. I put my hand over the end of my torch and switched on the light.

'Behold,' I said, 'before long we will see much along this path which will be of great interest.' And again, little did I know! Then, startlingly close at hand, came the cry of the hyena, followed immediately by the most appalling noise as though someone had got hold of one of our tins, and was bashing it against every hard object in the neighbourhood. Ng'wagu was crouched in the corner saying, '*Weeh, Weeh!*'

Daudi grasped a knobbed stick. Petro picked up a native axe. I pressed the button of the torch. It showed directly in front of us the old car pointing straight down the road. Then the light picked out a tawny animal as big as an Alsatian dog, careering round in the wildest fashion. Suddenly it paused, turned towards us, and we could see that it was a hyena with its head firmly stuck in the tin which had contained the rancid dripping.

Daudi started to shake with laughter. '*Kumbe*, Bwana, *mbisi*, the hyena, is caught in one of our traps.'

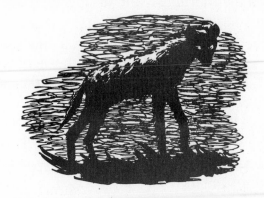

Ng'wagu's voice came from the back. 'What is happening, Bwana? What is happening? Tell me! Tell me!'

'*Hongo*,' started Daudi, but his words were interrupted as a most appalling clatter came from further down the road. The beam of light showed a figure on the ground struggling, and a kerosene tin continued to bang. I dashed across to the car, turned on the headlights, and there in a tunnel of light was Berenge struggling on the ground.

He was startled by the sudden noise which had come in the stillness of the night. This had changed to fear when he had fallen over the string. Then came the glaring, unexpected light of the car. To cap it all, the hyena suddenly bolted down the track blindly, its head firmly wedged in the tin. Berenge had struggled to his feet, managing to disentangle himself from the string and turn to run in panic when the hyena caught him behind the knees. Over they went together in a struggling mass – scavenger of the forest and witchdoctor. The struggle helped to knock the tin from the animal's mouth. With a strangled yelp it leapt off through the thornbush and disappeared down the path at an amazing speed.

I switched off the light. There was a crash and the danger cry, 'Weeh!' I switched on the lights again. Berenge had careered in the sudden darkness into a thornbush. Once again he was down. Again he struggled to his feet and disappeared round a corner of the track at speed. I was weak with laughter.

In the background old Ng'wagu kept saying, 'What is happening? Tell me. Tell me.'

Petro and Daudi told the story, interrupting it every now and then with gusts of laughter, but old Ng'wagu sat still, listening to every word of it. Then a slow smile came over his face. 'Should one who can turn himself into a hyena fear when another hyena bumps into him?'

'Kumbe, Great One,' I said, 'may it not be that Bernege is a fraud?'

'Heh,' nodded the old man, 'Bwana, my fear has gone. Truly the power of God is great, not only to put to flight those who are against Him, but also to bring comfort and laughter to those who would follow His path.'

'Truly,' I said, 'listen, and I will tell you the words of God's Book. There was one who followed God with all his heart. His name was Elisha. He heard that three great chiefs were going to fight against another great chief. They travelled through the desert on a road that was long and weary. Behold, before they had reached the place to which they wished to go, their supply of water failed for both man and beast. So they came to Elisha and asked him that he should pray to God that they might be helped.

'Elisha stood before them and said, "the Lord of Hosts, the God I serve, is a living God. Behold, I have a message for you from Him. Dig channels here, channels there, in this dry river-bed. These are the words of the Lord. Never a sign shall there be of wind or rain, but this river-bed shall fill with water, for you and yours, and your beasts to drink, but the Lord will not be content with that. He means to give you a victory."

'And next morning, in came water. Water filled the whole plains. Then they saw an army marching upon them. They called every man who could fight, to fight. They stood ready to defend their frontier. The storm broke, and the sun rose. The sunrise was reflected in the water so that it seemed from the enemies' side of the valley to be red as blood. "Blood," they cried, "the kings have fallen out with each other and have come to blows. *Kah,* let us smite them and take the spoil." They rushed in to the fight and were beaten.'

'*Hongo*,' said old Ng'wagu, 'Bwana, these are strong words. Surely God is of great strength, and shows it to those who go His way.'

'*Heeh,*' I replied, 'have we not seen it?'

At that moment, in the thornbush came once again the voice of the hyena,

'*Heh,*' said the old man, 'the voice of *mbisi* brings no more fear now. *Hongo*, it is only a short time before I arrive at the hospital. Bwana, you can work on my eyes with your little knife.'

5
Wild Safari

The door flew open. Daudi came in.

'Bwana,' he said, 'the children tell me that there is great sickness in the nose of your car. *Heh*, I would think that last night Berenge got caught in our traps going away and not coming. Behold, there is a big gash …'

I waited to hear no more but dashed through the door. There, underneath the car was a drying patch of rusty water. The radiator had a gaping hole in it. Only an axe could have made that twisted, unmendable hole. There was nothing for it. We would have to get a new radiator; this might take a month.

I turned around to Daudi.

'Is there any way that we can get to the train? It is most important that we get on with this safari, and get all this stuff to the station.'

Daudi scratched his head, 'There is the ancestor of vehicles here; it is surely the old one of all cars.'

Before long we were doing our best to fix up the old Mission car. It required both medicine and surgery. A jack under the back axle of that old bus, long ago dubbed "Methuselah", was a familiar sight. It had been old, unspeakably old, when I had first seen it years before. Petro was armed with a 2lb hammer, and to use his own words was 'just fixing things up a bit.'

I lay on the ground and pushed and kicked the back springs.

'Just a little bit more to the south, Bwana.'

I kicked.

'*Hodo*,' he cried, 'that'll do. You know, Bwana, the only time the brakes work in this old bus is when those centre bolts act as a brake, and then everything comes on at once.'

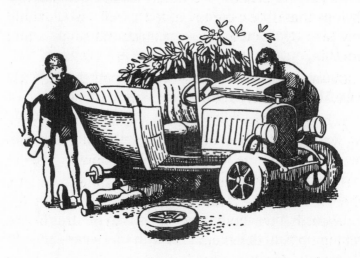

I pointed out that the back axle was still about an inch out of alignment, so we tightened up sundry nuts and bolts and set off on a trial run through the hospital grove of frangipani. Gingerly, I pushed the brakes. There was a fearful clatter.

'*Kah*,' grunted Petro, 'use the gears, Bwana. Don't try the brakes unless you've got to.'

Carefully, I pushed down the clutch and we discovered that second gear just didn't work; we had only first and top.

'I say, Petro, how does Bibi, the Jungle Nurse, get on when she drives this awful thing?'

Petro laughed. '*Hongo*, Bwana, you know they tell me that when she gets into a car that's got brakes, she doesn't know how to drive it!'

Then we found that there was no reverse gear in the car either, so we had rather an exhausting time pushing it round, moving it a foot at a time. At last, in the early afternoon, we were loaded up and it was obvious that if we were to get to the railway, we could only take Ng'wagu a mile or two on his safari. I told him this.

'Bwana,' he said, 'if there is someone to lead me, I will gladly walk, if in front of me there is hope of light.'

'*Yoh*,' said Daudi, as I waved goodbye to Petro, 'Ng'wagu has the best of this safari. He travels only to the place where the road goes up and down.'

He rolled his eyes as I warned him against splinters, when I noticed he braced his bare feet against the floorboards. We both saw with alarm the smoke welling up between them.

With a crash we arrived in top gear as the road levelled out and swung past the village. Berenge's mud-and-wattle house looked very ordinary. A skinny hen scratched industriously where last night the sinister figure of the witchdoctor had stalked.

The old car bumped noisily over the sun-cracked earth. Ng'wagu clung to the side, his face set. We ground our way over plains, through a palm-tree swamp, with a clutter of goats and fat-tailed sheep claiming every patch of shade.

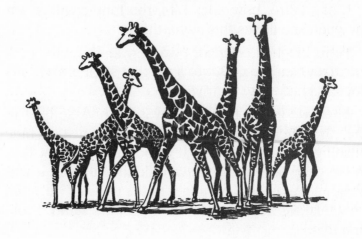

A bend in the road brought us face to face with a group of great golden-crested cranes. They flapped up into the hot air heavily, and not a minute further on, seven silent giraffes looked mildly at us as we swirled past in our dust cloud. Before us the red road, incredibly rough, seemed to stand on end.

'Ng'wagu,' I yelled above the engine's noise, 'it is here that you get down and walk.'

The old man shuffled to his feet. '*Yoh*, Bwana, it is better to walk. *Kah*,' he rubbed his skinny flanks feelingly.

Daudi grinned. 'Truly, yours is the smoothest safari. The Bwana and I must travel in this kerosene tin on wheels.'

'*Kwaheri*, goodbye,' we cried as we drove on and watched the old blind man jogging along in our dust.

Ahead, red gashes in the jungle indicated the turbulent course of the road we were to travel.

I found it necessary to perform like an organist on the pedals, and swing the gear lever from top to low gear in the most disconcerting way.

Above the noise, Daudi shouted. 'Petro says she's got a grand engine.' His voice lacked conviction, warranted I felt when I noted a certain independence of action between engine and body, to such an extent that that 'grand engine' seemed as though it might go on alone, and leave us behind! Daudi gripped more firmly the portions of the wooden body of the car that were whole. A piece of three-ply where the windscreen was supposed to meet the dashboard had a fascinating habit of jumping up and coming down in approximately the same place again, but I was too busy to hold that in place.

We screamed round a bend in low gear and I banged the door for the twentieth time.

'You need three hands to drive this car,' I yelled, 'one for the gears, one for the steering, and one to bang the door.'

Daudi clung to the door and said nothing.

The road swung into position where there was a drop of hundreds of feet on the unfenced side. You can imagine my feelings when one hand went to the gears and the other ached to slam the door which swung wide with a view of a precipice below.

We climbed the steep ascent and the old car was blowing steam of a rich brown colour, which swirled in, almost obscuring our view. We stopped jerkily, Daudi leaping out and thrust stones under the wheels. With the engine running, we filled the radiator from a dented petrol tin and then, turning her off to cool, I got underneath with a screw wrench and a 2lb hammer and rearranged the transmission! I stood up again, shaking off dust and removing grease from my face with a piece of cotton waste.

'We've got to rely on the gears, Daudi. The brakes might skid us over to one side and...' I looked from that drop to the sheer wall and shuddered.

Daudi rolled his eyes and swung the crank handle. Methuselah coughed and condescended to start, as the track ran downhill. We swerved uncomfortably fast round a steep corner. Two hundred yards ahead of us was a herd of cattle and sheep and goats, completely blocking the steepest part of the hill.

'The horn won't work!' I shouted.

'Could you hear it if it did, Bwana?' Daudi yelled back.

Apparently the noise of the old car was most effective. The startled herd scattered and we bounded through.

Daudi's mouth was wide open. '*Kah*, Bwana. I thought, "Surely, we will have meat with our porridge tonight!"'

At the bottom of the hill was a welcome straight, flat stretch. We had travelled perhaps a hundred yards along this when an explosion from the front tyre coincided with a mulish tug on the wheel in my hands. We swayed dizzily. The steering-wheel just seemed to be an ornament as the blow-out swung us almost on to our side.

'Yah,' said Daudi, scrambling over the door, 'if that had happened a mile back…'

We looked at the road along the side of the hill and thanked God. Daudi was rubbing a bump on the back of his head.

'Bwana,' he said, 'it would be a good thing to bring people who have no fear of death down that road. *Kah,* this would be the place to bring them that they might learn. *Hongo* …' He lapsed into speculation.

'It's only six miles to the railway station, Daudi, but there's another one of those to climb, and another descent before we get there.'

We found that the spare tyre was punctured and the tube looked largely perished. Finally, in desperation we stuffed the blown-out tyre with grass.

It was late afternoon by the time we had things in order again for the road. We were all covered with dust and sweat. The tepid water from the kerosene tin had a strong flavour of paraffin, but tasted very sweet to our dry throats.

The 'grand engine' seemed to be having a spell, for although each of us cranked until his arms were tired, she wouldn't start. So we pushed until Methuselah moved slowly forward. I let in the clutch and then suddenly, with a roar, the engine burst into life. Daudi stumbled and then, running like a hare, leapt over the tail-board for he knew that, once started, we didn't dare to stop. He crawled over the back and shook his head, shouting above the din.

'*Kah,* Bwana, what a safari!'

Night came down suddenly. Long grass crowded over the road. Overhead were ghostly trees. Dim huts, and the eyes of animals and night-birds, seemed to spring up out of the night. At last the great hill down to the railway station loomed up. We were negotiating a very narrow road with a deep black chasm on the far side. The gears screamed again as we changed down and then the headlights cut out. Darkness hit us like a black wall. I groped for my torch, clinging desperately to the bucking steering-wheel, and shone it through the place where there would normally have been a windscreen. I managed somehow to keep on that narrow road.

There was just sufficient light to show us where to go and then the headlights decided to come on again. A few seconds later and our hectic safari might have

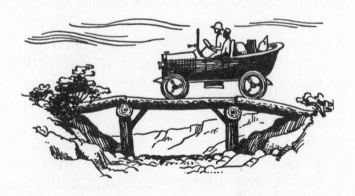

ended in tragedy. On two wheels we swung round a bend. The tree, the bank and the ditch all missed us.

We rattled over a precarious bridge and then we saw the train half a mile away, standing in the station. We swept through the native town and the lights failed again, but there was nothing to stop us in the last hundred yards.

We scrambled on to the railway track, dashing to and from the old car laden with boxes. With a sigh I pushed the last box on to the train, when the Indian station-master, who had watched with interest, said, 'There is no call for haste, sir. The train is delayed here some two hours.'

Daudi looked solemnly at me and said in Chigogo, 'Truly, Bwana, it was the dog who hurried who had the blind pups.'

In three languages I wrote a note which I tied to the steering-wheel of Methuselah – *'Please return, preferably by towing.'*

Some days later I received in Petro's careful handwriting:

To Bwana:

I am well through the goodness of God. I trust you too are well. The news of our safari is that we returned with nimbleness somewhat. Half journey up the hill the steering-wheel came apart from the floorboards. It was in my hands by itself. Our fortune was that we travelled at slow speed and also uphill. By skill and many strengths I managed well to slow down and pull up, but had fear again when the brakes gave refusal to hold and car and we began to roll back downhill. Fears were may but were lessened by a slight bank and there we came to rest uprightly with thanks.

Before attempt to climb over last hill we supported steering-column with a forked stick of strength and much rope used like bandage.

Many thanks to God we are home in whole skin.

I remain, dear Sir and Doctor,

Your obedient servant,

PETRO BIN MUSA.'

6
Glass Eye

The train had meandered comfortably along through the night, and here, in the early morning, was Dodoma township. Carefully we unloaded all the baggage and then I heard Daudi's voice behind me:

'Bwana, you see the one coming towards us? He is Yacobo upon whom you did much work. Has he not one eye that sees, and one that does not? *Kumbe,*

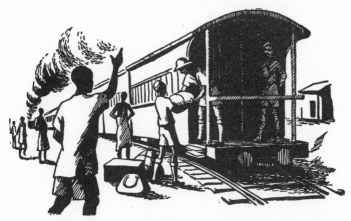

and to look at him, is it not hard to tell which eye is which?'

Yacobo had come up by this time and gripped my hand.

'*Mbukwa*, Bwana.'

'*Mbukwa*,' I replied. 'It is many days since I saw you.'

'*Eheeh*, Bwana, and days full of happiness they are, for you worked with great strength to help my face. Once I had shame because of my one eye, but now that I have three, *hongo,* all is well!'

'*Yoh*, Yacobo, three eyes?'

'*Eheeh*, Bwana, one that sees, two that do not. One that is my day eye, *hongo*, and another that is my night eye. It rest in the daytime in its small bottle.'

Daudi and I both laughed.

'*Kumbe*, it certainly has made a change in your appearance since we fixed that eye.'

Daudi nodded. '*Eheeh*, Bwana. Do you remember? It was almost at this spot near the railway station, where we first met Yacobo.'

'*Eheeh*, I remember that, but give me food for my memory, Yacobo. I forget the details of the story of how your trouble started.'

The train from which we had alighted whistled shrilly, and moved out of Dodoma station. Two small African boys dressed in the smallest amount of cloth tied around their middle stopped to watch incuriously. The skinny goats they were herding took even less notice. Yacobo pointed towards them with his chin.

'I was like that, Bwana. My age was perhaps eight or nine. I was in charge of my father's goats when all my trouble started. I had to keep them from the weeds that were poisonous and find food for them in the days of dryness. *Heh*, Bwana, it was much work, and as I drove them through the thornbush, the limb of one of the trees swung back and hit me in the face. One of the thorns...'

He reached up to break off a vicious-looking specimen from a nearby tree; it was three inches long and hard as wire.

'One of these thorns, Bwana, went right through my eyelid into my eye. *Heeh,* the pain was great but I thought little of it. It had happened before. When I went home, I told my father about it.'

'"*Hongo*," he said, 'we must have medicine for that." So he pulled back my eyelid and licked the eyeball. He also took medicine from a gourd that had been given him by Ng'oma, the witchdoctor. *Koh*, that night the eye was sore and the next day it was swollen. Behold, soon came *ichiligala*, an eye ulcer. Each day it became worse and I saw less and less until darkness came upon that eye. *Kumbe*, Bwana, and the pain... *Yoh*, the pain... One night I lay at home on my cowskin in the house and groaned. The smoke from the fire irritated my eye. The flies wouldn't leave me alone. Bwana, *koh*, there was pain. That was the worst of it, and afterwards the redness left the eye. But, Bwana, the sight was gone. Behold, through the years my eye had been blind and many were those who shuddered when they looked at it.'

'*Eheeh*, Yacobo. Truly, it was an organ of small joy. *Hongo*, I remember your coming to the hospital and how I read very hard in my medical books, for it was a work I had never before done.'

Daudi nodded. '*Kumbe*, Bwana, we prayed with strength and operated with hands that shook a little. Remember?'

I nodded.

'*Yoh*,' smiled Yacobo. 'However your hands shook, Bwana, you succeeded in taking out what remained where my eye should have been. *Koh*, it was no good to me. You gave me an eye just the same colour as the one that works…One that I could put in and take out.'

He suited the action to the words. Holding his glass eye in front of me, he said:

'Of course, I couldn't see with it but it took from my face the cause of shame.'

I smiled and nodded.

'*Kumbe*, and even these days when I meet strangers and show them this eye, they have great amazement. Truly, it has given me a chance to tell them what they couldn't understand otherwise. I've told them that when you try to look out of your glass eye you see nothing. If you choose to look with your glass eye, you walk in darkness. But when you look with your real eye, then you see things as they are and I told them the words of God's Book which says, "This is the judgment that has come into the world, that men loved darkness rather than light, because their deeds were evil,"' and I told them that many men choose to go their own way and not God's way, and they look

70

with their own eyes, and not with God-given eyes. Do I not show them that if I walk round the place looking with my glass eye only, my hand over the good one, *yoh!* I get into trouble; I fall, bump into things? If I go round the place looking with my good eye, then I follow the right path. This is the message that I pass on with my new glass eye...'

'*Hongo,* Yacobo, these are words of truth,' nodded Daudi, 'words you must tell to an old man named Ng'wagu. He is coming to hospital that he also may receive light again into eyes that see less than we do at clouded midnight when the moon sleeps.'

'He will be led by the hand, Yacobo. Give him food and also show him the way to Buigiri Hospital. I will be working there for many days.'

Yacobo nodded. '*He hee!* Bwana, it is already as good as done.'

7

Blind School

I stood on the veranda of the C.M.S. Buigiri Hospital and looked at the crowd of people waiting for medicine.

'*Koh*, Daudi, at two minutes each it will take us five hours to cope with this crowd!'

My African helper looked at the people grouped around in the shade, some clutching gourds containing millet seed, their 'thank you' for the medicine. One old man with his leg tied up with an incredibly dirty rag had a thin chicken tied to his toe. A young woman, with a very sick baby on her knee, sat huddled against the wall, nervously fingering a charm round her neck. I wrinkled my nose, which told me a story of mixed scents: of goat, of antiseptic, of wood smoke and of frangipani.

Daudi had been counting the patients.

'*Hongo*, Bwana, your words are true. There are more than a hundred and fifty people here, with more diseases than there are in the book's index.'

'Come on then, let us work.'

We got solidly on with the task, and before long there was a noisy clanking of medicine glasses; a hissing of breath as a strong African nurse rubbed liniment with vigour; a dispenser was most busy with an eye-dropper, while Daudi was hard at it with a syringe and a collection of small bottles.

From where I sat, listening to an African's chest with my stethoscope, I could see a cloud of dust, brown against the blue hills. As this came closer, I saw a lorry swaying precariously. It turned up the path

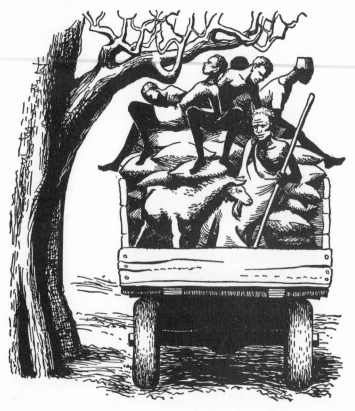

towards the hospital. As it came closer, I could see its Somalilander driver with yellow turban, a purple shirt and green velveteen trousers. The vehicle was loaded high with bags of millet on which was perched a group of African men and small boys, ducking as the vehicle swung under the limbs of a baobab tree, to pull up before the hospital. Wedged against the tail-board was a bearded billy goat, more apparent to the nose than the eye, almost pushing old Ng'wagu on to the floor.

I got up to help the old man to his feet.

'*Yoh*,' he said, 'Bwana, *heeeh*, this is a way of sorrow to travel.'

A gourd of water was brought for him to drink and drops were put into his eyes.

The sun was blazingly hot overhead when I gave the last dose of medicine. Ng'wagu lay asleep on the concrete floor, his head resting on his arm.

'Bwana,' said Daudi, 'let him rest and later this afternoon we will have words with him, after food has comforted his stomach.'

It was *saa kumi*, the tenth hour, if you tell the time Swahili fashion, four o'clock if you prefer it by more orthodox means, when a cup of tea was brought to me. I ordered another to be poured out for Ng'wagu. He was sitting on a form, looking sightlessly over the plains.

'Great One,' I said, 'would you care to moisten your tongue?'

The old man drank deeply and gratefully.

'*Assante*, Bwana. *Heh*, it is with joy that I sit here in the cool and yet, Bwana, with sadness. My nose tells me many things but I long to see my own country with my own eyes.'

I felt a touch on my arm. 'Bwana, come over and have a look at the Blind School.'

I looked up to see Paolo, a blind teacher. He moved unhesitatingly round the room, avoiding things in a way that amazed me.

'Paolo, I have here a sick one. He, too, would visit your school. He, too, walks in darkness but would seek the light.'

Paolo moved round to where Ng'wagu was sitting.

'Come,' he said, 'and hear the words of the place where the sting is taken out of darkness.'

One blind man gripped the arm of the other. They travelled down the steps, along the path to a mud brick building where a dozen blind folk, men and

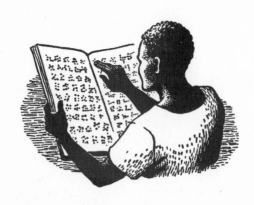

boys, were busily engaged in making baskets, while one of them with a Braille book was reading at a great speed with his fingers. On a table lay sheets of Braille writing. Behind it, neatly arranged along the wall was a carpenter's bench and then a neat pile of mats and a handloom, and a pile of other devices foreign to me.

Paolo came to my side, seeming to sense where I was though his eyes were obviously sightless.

'Bwana, welcome to our school.'

I was about to reply, when the words seemed to dry up in my throat. I tapped Paolo on the shoulder gently.

'Over there, the big fellow in the corner! Surely that's Meshak?'

The African beside me nodded.

'*Eheh*, Bwana, it is indeed.'

It was as though someone had thrown a film on a screen. The whole story of that African seemed to surge back into my mind. Time seemed to go back ten years in as many seconds.

The C.M.S. Boys' School headmaster had bailed me up under a mango tree.

'There's a man I want you to see here, Doctor. He's rather a sad story. Once he was one of our most skilful carpenters that came out of the school.'

'That so? What's his name?'

'Meshak. From the point of view of his trade, he was one of the best people we ever had. But somehow he just wasn't interested in the biggest things that the school had to offer. He passed his examinations and then just disappeared into the blue. We heard of him from time to time. It appeared that he was working with some Indians and getting good money, but the more cash he got, the more beer his wife brewed and the more slovenly he became. Then he just faded completely out of our knowledge until this morning when I saw one of those pathetic processions that are all too common here. In front was a small boy. I recognised him. He was Meshak's child. Behind him, his mother, leading by a stick her husband, on her head a basket with their provisions and all their worldly goods. He wore a great broad felt hat and was dressed in tatters. He groaned and groaned with one hand over his eyes. I had one peep at these and realised it was a job for you.'

'What happened to him? The usual thing?'

'Yes. Witchdoctors again.'

'What? Do you mean to tell me, after all he learned here he went into the jungle and let those fellows chew up bark and leaves and rubbish of that sort, and spit it into his eyes from their filthy mouths?'

'Well, have a look at him. You'll soon tell the tale. It looks very much like it to me.'

I walked across the dry river-bed to where, under a thornbush, sat Meshak, his hand over his eyes, muttering in his misery.

'*Mbukwa*. May I help you?'

Meshak groaned. 'My trouble is a very great one.'

I bent over and attempted to turn back the eyelid. His eyes were in a dreadful condition, but the groan changed almost to a scream. His nerves were on edge for he must have suffered unspeakable things. He had been walking five days and he had got to the stage when malaria had muddled his mind. The complete tangle of his thoughts had brought him almost to breaking point. In the shade I managed to separate his eyelids. There was the horrible sight of an eye utterly inflamed. It didn't take me long to make the diagnosis. We *might* – there was a very big *might* about it – manage to save his sight to a small degree, but there was real doubt about even that. He almost certainly was hopelessly blinded.

Meshak put his hand on the side of his head and in a pitiful voice said, 'Bwana, I followed the way of my own will. I turned my back on the words of God. I followed the ways of the tribe. *Hehe*, look what's happened, Bwana. Everything is dark, agonisingly dark. Bwana, let me die.'

'You must come to the hospital, Meshak. Behold, I will give you medicine to quieten your pain.'

My memories of ten years before were broken as suddenly Meshak stumbled to his feet and came across to me.

'Bwana,' he said, *'kah,* Bwana.' He gripped my hands in a way that hurt.

'*Hongo*, and behold, the medicines have at no time helped your eyes, my friend?'

He shook his head. '*Ng'o*, but, Bwana, I have learnt many things with my fingers. Can I not read the paper with little lumps on it? Can I not work with my hands, and am I not still a good carpenter? Behold, can I not also make baskets and mats? *Kumbe!* I have ceased to worry about my eyes.'

He bent his head somewhat because he was well over six feet, and said quietly in my ear, 'Bwana, I thank God for my blindness. Had I kept my eyesight, *heh*, would I then have gone the ways of God? Was I not following fast in the paths of the devil until, Bwana … until those days?'

From across the room came the voice of the old blind man, Ng'wagu.

'Bwana, behold, I wish to move on to the place where the medicine will be given me. Have I not walked very many miles? Have I not been bruised for many more in these cars? It is a matter for speed, Bwana.'

'Who is this?' breathed Meshak. 'Bwana, what are his words?'

'He is an old one of the tribe. He has the disease we call cataracts. He has travelled many miles to come to the hospital.'

Meshak moved across to the old man. 'Have courage and patience, Great One, the Bwana will help you. Great is his skill in the removal of darkness.'

A stool was brought and the old man sat down.

'*Hongo*, Great One, he has done very much for me. Berenge made medicines that destroyed my eyes. But the Bwana, oh, how he helped.'

'*Kumbe,*' said the old man, 'tell me the story.'

'At the time of the evening porridge, I will tell you these words. The Bwana also will strengthen my memory with his own words.'

I watched the blind carpenter's wife pounding millet, separating the husks from the grain in a large, flat basket and then grinding the flour between two stones. Soon great clay pots were steaming, crows flew raggedly overhead and the sun set as I watched blind folk walking the hard trodden paths with amazing certainty.

'Bwana,' said Daudi, 'there would be joy if you would eat the food of the village.'

So a stool was brought and I sat eating *wugali*, porridge, with Meshak, Daudi, Paolo and old Ng'wagu.

Mosquitoes hummed round. On the hill behind the house a hyena laughed. The smell of wood smoke and the soft warmness of the night called aloud for the 'round the fire' story-telling that Africans dearly love.

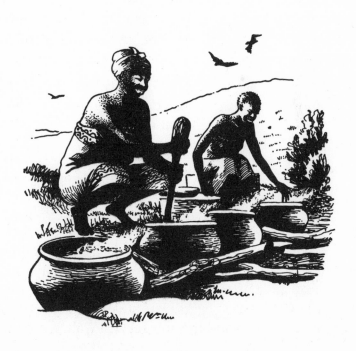

8

Firelight Memories

Meshak sat with his head forward, the firelight showing up some of the white hairs in the close-cropped curls of his head. His fingers grasped a pebble which he rolled ceaselessly between their tips.

'*Yoh*,' he said. 'In the days when I came to the C.M.S. Hospital many harvests ago I had despair, black despair. There was pain that held me. I could not escape it. It was like fire, a slow fire that burnt into me. Then I seemed to hear a voice in my ear: 'And may not fire be quenched?'

'*Heh*, my thoughts travelled this path. A gourd full of water will quickly put out a fire. I could do this to the fire that burnt within me. My fingers touched the hunting-knife strapped to my side, here was the answer!'

'*Hongo!*' Daudi's voice came out of the gloom. 'But I too saw your fingers and saw your hand toy with that knife and start to draw it. *Yoh*! I grabbed your arm and fought, while the boy with the broken wrist ran to call the Bwana.'

I broke in. '*Kumbe*, and I remember it was a night of thunder and of sudden lightning. A small boy, one arm in plaster of Paris, the other clasping his pyjama trousers, stood breathlessly outside my door.

"Bwana! Bwana! *Upesi*, quickly, great danger!'

'*Hongo*, how I ran, listening as I did so to the wind sighing through the cornstalks. Behind the hospital, *mbisi*, the hyena, laughed horribly. *Hongo*, my flesh crept on my bones. It was a night of evil. Through the *ibolulu*, the courtyard, I ran and into the men's ward. *Yoh*, every patient was sitting up, full of fright, looking towards the corner bed.

'There, Daudi, you were struggling in the dim light. Suddenly there was a flash and a clatter, and a hunting-knife fell to the floor.'

Meshak's voice interrupted my story.

'*Heh*, Bwana, you arrived just in time. *Koh*, how I fought for that knife! I wanted to use it. Life was *bwete,* hopeless.'

The flickering flame of the fire showed up old Ng'wagu squatting on a stool, his head in his hands.

'*Koh*,' he breathed, 'what did you do?'

'*Hongo*,' said Meshak, leaning back on his stool, his hands behind his head, 'what could I do? Behold, one held my arm with strength and twisted it until I dropped the knife and then, Bwana, you spoke to me. But your voice had no anger in it. You talked of my eyes and my troubles and I had no words of reply.

'I screamed in rage and despair and I used strong words to bring anger to your heart, and from there to your lips; but *koh*, Bwana, none came. Within me was fear, fear of darkness. Life was empty. Were not my eyes ruined? Before me was nothing but darkness, thick darkness and despair. *Hongo*, and I heard the message of the drums, the message of the wind through the corn and the rumble of the thunder in the hills. Then shrill came the voice of the hyena, and I knew I was bewitched and bound with strong spells. *Kah*, Bwana, I wished with strong desire to go to be with my ancestors. *Yoh*, but Bwana, still you spoke softly.

'"Meshak, because you're in darkness, because of what has happened to your eyes, is that all that matters? Is there no other part of you worth living for?"

'*Heh*, I tore at the hands that held me and screamed, "Let me go! Let me go!"'

Ng'wagu was taut. His sightless eyes peered at Meshak, his lips moving speechlessly, his hand locked on the knob of his stick.

Meshak spat into the fire. 'Bwana, your words were these, "Many of your tribe, when they feel as you do, do they not die? Do they not let their spirits sift from their bodies as a woman lets flour run through her fingers? Will you not do the same?" "*Kah*," I groaned, "Bwana, I want to! I want to! But I can't, I can't! There's something that holds me!"

'Bwana, your hand was on my shoulder. "*Heh*," you agreed, "I know what holds you. It is fear, Meshak. You have stood outside your house at night. You have seen the camp fire. You have heard the stories of the tribe. You have seen the meals prepared and then the fire burns low. The coals glow; they become white with ash. You see a red glimpse now and again, and then the fire is out. But life does not go like that. There is something after the last glow has gone out of the body. That is the soul, the part of you that matters to God, the part of you that never dies. You can't kill the soul with a knife."

Kah, Bwana and I had great fear at your words for I knew they were true. You let these thoughts sink in and then you said, "Meshak, you have played the fool in letting your eyes be ruined by the medicines of Berenge. Do not play the fool twice." "Hongo," I cried, "what shall I do then?" Your words came quietly, Bwana. They stand out in my memory as does the Braille writing on its paper. "Your eyes are dull but there is still light available for your soul. Why not ask God to come into your life, to bring light into the eyes of your soul so that you may live and have the Light of Life inside you?" There were other words, Bwana, but these remained in my mind with strength.'

'*Hongo*,' said old Ng'wagu hoarsely, moving his toes up and down in the dust, 'and did the Bwana bring light again to your eyes?'

Daudi's voice came in reply. 'Listen, Great One, larger things than this occurred. At cock-crow next morning Meshak and I had many words, and then we walked to the Bwana's house and greeted him. Then Meshak said, "Bwana, I have not slept. I lay there, and as I lay, calm came over me somehow and I felt that what I had planned in my frenzy was a way of small wisdom. It was walking into more unknown darkness."'

Meshak got to his feet and walked across to where some firewood was neatly piled, picked up a log and with the utmost precision placed it on the fire. It seemed incredible that the man doing what he had just done could be blind.

'*Kumbe*, Bwana,' he said, 'when Daudi and I had been talking earlier that morning, he had told me of one like myself, named Petro, an impulsive man. Jesus said to him, "Follow Me," and Petro followed. *Koh*, he made his mistakes. Behold, once he denied that he even knew his Master when a woman laughed. *Heh*, I thought, I would not do that but then I saw it wasn't easy to follow Jesus. Behold, Daudi made me understand that it is not just a matter of words, of saying that you agree to His teaching, if you would follow His way. Behold, it was not just a matter of sitting, but if I were to follow Him it was a matter of learning to see with my fingers, to work with my hands so that my life would not be *bwete*, worthless. These were the words, Bwana, spoken harvests ago, which are alive in my mind still.'

'*Hongo*,' said Paolo, the blind teacher, speaking for the first time. '*Yoh*, how he worked, Bwana. His fingers are now as active as mine. He reads with speed. He's a good carpenter. He...'

'*Koh*,' came Ng'wagu's deep voice. 'He walks with comfort in darkness while I ... *Eeeh*.' He sighed.

'*Eheeh*,' lauged Meshak, 'the darkness will go when the Bwana works with his knife, and you will live comfortably in light with your ordinary eyes. *Kumbe*, Great One, when light comes to them do not, however, forget the inner eyes.'

9

On Safari to Mvumi

Slowly Ng'wagu stood up. 'I shall travel on my feet, Bwana, to finish this safari.'

''*Heh*, but it's twenty miles, Ng'wagu.'

He ran his toes through the dust and said, '*Heh*, Bwana, I can feel the way it goes. I, who have walked in darkness for many days can find a path with my feet, where many cannot see it with their eyes. But, Bwana, I do not see the thorns. *Yoh!*' He puckered up his nose. 'However, thorns are better than to travel crash! To travel – *hooh!* – in that.' He pointed disdainfully to where the hospital truck stood with its engine running, made two dramatic poses and caressed the appropriate portion of his anatomy. '*Heh*, let me walk.'

'Right, go your own way, Ng'wagu. Our safari is nearly finished, and it will be tomorrow or the day after that we will have you in bed preparing for the day when, by the goodness of God, and with His hand upon mine, sight will come back.'

'*Heh*, Bwana, there are days when I think that it will never come – this light that you speak of. For so many days it has been darkness, darkness, nothing but darkness. *Hongo*, but I have hope, a small hope that grows, Bwana.'

'*Alu! Ng'hubita* - I set out!'

He plodded off down the track. Through a haze of red dust I could see his forlorn figure moving on along the path, his stick questing in front of him. His mind was set on one thing – sight.

Daudi had filled the radiator and blown up the tyres. With a multitude of *kwaheris*, goodbyes, we set out. The road wound through the jungle. Small monkeys 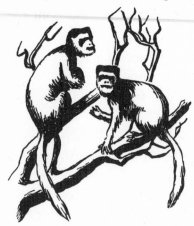 gibbered at us and crows cawed discordantly. We careered down a sharp-cut bank into a dry river-bed. Driving the truck crab fashion, we negotiated it and with a skidding of wheels climbed the other side, to see before us in the distance the old man's figure moving resolutely on. Then came a grinding crash. We passed him, Daudi shouting encouragement, and had negotiated two more rivers when suddenly the engine roared but the truck came to an uneasy standstill.

'*Kah*,' said Daudi sitting beside me, 'Bwana, that is another axle gone. Why did we have this car repaired and brought from Makutopora? Now we will lie in the dust. We will have oil dripping all over us and no opportunity to dodge.'

This gloomy prophecy was only too true. Fortunately we had a spare axle, and proceeded to fit it. This is no easier than it sounds. We were groping with an ingenious contrivance that looks like an elongated corkscrew, when the old blind man came up.

'*Yah,*' he said with a smile on his face, 'behold, *ilawaliwa*, the tortoise, walks with more speed than *sungura*, the rabbit.'

'*Yah,*' said Daudi his mouth half full of oil, 'did you ever hear *sungura*, the rabbit, roar like this machine?'

The old man walked on, one foot on the concave side of the path, the other in its centre.

'*Chokwiwoni*, we will see one another,' he laughed and plodded on into the glaring heat.

After two hours of struggle, Daudi and I looked much the same colour. We crawled out from underneath the old bus, looked at one another and laughed. There was no water, so, sitting on part of a copy of the *Tanganyika Standard*, and wiping my hands on another part of the same valuable journal, we proceeded on our way, and came to a village where there were some Indian and Arab shops. Sulimani, my friend in a score of emergencies, seeing my plight, supplied me with the appropriate in the way of hot water and blue, very alkaline, soap. I soon got back to my normal colour.

'Sulimani, did you see an old man, blind, walking this way?'

'*Heh, heh*,' nodded the Indian, 'I put him on the path to Mvumi Hospital. He walked like one who has a desire to arrive.'

'*Heh*, will we not operate on his eyes before long?'

Sulimani nodded his head. 'This is a work of great value.'

I thanked him for his help, wiped the grease off the steering-wheel and then found that the old truck would not start. Thirty or forty small boys proceeded to push us along the very flat road. We went past shops, the mud-brick Muslim mosque, then down a slight slope. I let in the clutch, and with a roar we were on our way again. I waved my thanks to the cheering small boys and settled down to the last eight miles of the safari.

We climbed a hill. Coming in our direction along the road ahead of us was a tall figure.

'*Kah*, Daudi, surely that is not Ng'wagu?'

Daudi taughtened, and whistled quietly through his teeth.

'*Kah*, Bwana, this is Ng'oma, the witchdoctor, the relation of Berenge who has given us all the trouble. See, he wears the head-dress of a witchdoctor and the ornaments on his wrists.'

As we came closer I could see, wound round his head, a cowskin. In each hand he held a great gourd with a stopper carved to represent a man's head. As we stopped he put down his gourd and stalked up. I wondered what was coming next, then his hand came out.

'Bwana,' he said, '*mbukwa*.'

'*Mbukwa*,' I said, grasping both his hands in mine, in the ceremonial handshake.

'Bwana, I have seen an old man of the tribe walking along the path past my house. He walks with strength, and as I met him on the road, he told me you have strong medicine for eyes. Look even now into my eyes, Great One. One gives such pain that sleep is gone. It burns.'

The sun was westering. In the mellow light I could see that one eye was definitely and uncomfortably swollen.

'Is it as though you had sand in your eye, O Ng'oma?' I asked.

'*Heh*, Bwana, but behold it itches and burns, and I dare not look into the light for the pain is there. Bwana, I have fear.'

'Bwana, the medicines of the Waganga are not strong to help the troubles of the eyes,' said Daudi.

I raised my eyebrows, not trusting myself to comment.

A half-smile came over the witchdoctor's face. 'Bwana, be generous with me. Give me this medicine for my eyes.'

'I'd be happy to do that.'

Then a most unusual thing happened. Ng'oma looked at me and said, 'Truly you could only do that. Behold, have I not the words?'

Daudi and I looked at each other, wondering what was coming next. To our amazement the witchdoctor started in the local language to recite the Lord's Prayer. This he did word-perfectly, and then said with a cunning look:

'You see, Bwana, I have the words. Are they not very strong medicine?'

'Listen, Ng'oma, that is wrong. Those are the words of a child speaking to his father. They're the words that Jesus Christ, the Great One, told us to pray when we are members of God's family. But, behold, did He not turn and say to them, "you are of your father, the devil?" Be careful to whom you pray, therefore, O Ng'oma, when you say "Our Father." You do not speak to God unless you become a member of His family, and, remember, a child obeys his father.'

'*Heeheeh*,' nodded Daudi.

'*Hongo*,' said Ng'oma, 'am I not one of His people?'

I shook my head. 'The things that you knew were right and have not done, these things God calls *sin* and sin is a strong wall between you and God. It is only Jesus Christ, God's Son, who can break down that wall and make peace between you and God.'

'*Heheeh*,' said Daudi, 'the Bwana's words are truth.'

'It is useless to mumble words. God says, "repent," which means change the whole of your mind about your work, your living, the way you treat people. Change your mind completely and then follow your mind with your feet (He calls this conversion), so that your actions reflect your thoughts. Ask Him to forgive you, then live your life His way.'

'*Hongo*,' said Ng'oma slowly, 'I thought that saying these words was all that was necessary, that they were a spell to make people do what I want.'

'*Uh, uh*, it is altogether more. It is a life to live, not just words to say. Come, get up with us into the truck and I will take you to the hospital and make medicine for your eyes.'

We moved on. The sky was beginning to redden with the sunset. We drove up a long, gently sloping hill. On the crest of it was a figure moving along with a stick in his hand. Slowly we came up behind him. The old man stood on the hill, looking with his hand shading his eyes into the great red globe which was the setting sun. I stood behind him.

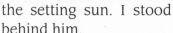

'*Yoh,* Ng'wagu, the tortoise at the very end of the safari. You are now within sight of the hospital.'

'Bwana,' he said, peering at the setting sun, 'it's red, the only light that comes to me is the colour of blood.' A shiver went through his frame.

The orb dipped behind the hill. You could see it disappearing slowly.

The old man said, 'Bwana, even that light has gone. It's darkness.'

'*Hongo*, and tomorrow, will not the sun rise?'

'*Heh*, Bwana.' He nodded.

'Will not the light come?'

'*Heh*, Bwana.' He nodded again.

'Have faith, therefore, about the light and your eyes.'

The old man's hand groped out towards me, touched my shoulder, moved down to my elbow. He held my hand.

'Bwana, it is this hand, these fingers that will bring back sight to me perhaps.'

I looked at my hands, coated with grease, the nails a far from professional sight.

'Great One, I also think of another hand, the palm of which holds a scar. It was that hand that brought light to my soul. That was the hand of God himself. He did a thing no other hand could do.'

'Bwana,' said the old man, 'tell me of this.'

Ng'oma, the witchdoctor, in the back of the car said, 'Behold, I too would hear these words.'

10

Witchdoctor Patient

'Pump up the pressure lamp, Daudi. Now place it on the window-sill above Ng'oma's head.'

'*Kah*,' said the witchdoctor in alarm, 'it hisses at me!'

'Sit quietly,' I ordered, adjusting a head mirror.

The intense white light flashed into the dark face before me. Both his eyes closed almost with a snap.

'*Hongo*,' my voice was sharp, 'do not squeeze up your eye.'

From behind me came a whisper. '*Kumbe*, fear is the heart of the man who has pain.'

Ng'oma opened his lids a fraction. '*Yoh*,' he gasped, 'the light glares!'

With dropper poised Daudi was ready and local anaesthetic went into both eyes.

'*Ukkkk!*' he yelled, nearly knocking me over as he struggled to his feet in panic. '*Ehhh*, the pain!'

'*Heh*,' said Daudi in disgust. 'It is small pain only.'

'He did not say "*ukkkk!*" when he spat medicine into my eyes,' said a deep voice in the shadow.

'Come,' grunted Daudi, 'open wide that more drops, green ones, may be put in.'

'Green ones!' gulped Ng'oma, 'will not they cause pain?" Why...?'

'*Kah*,' I said, 'you must trust yourself into my hands. The first medicine stops pain, the second shows where the trouble is and I see the grit in your eye like the deep green of grass round a well in dry country.'

Ng'oma's eyes slowly opened. I shone the light in.

He smiled. 'Truly, Bwana, that is strong medicine. Even now the pain has gone.'

He would have got up and gone home if Daudi had not grasped his shoulders and said firmly, 'The pain, O witchdoctor, has gone truly, but the cause of it remains.'

Leaning forward, I held the eye open.

I picked up the battered alarm-clock we used for taking pulses.

'There, Daudi, set it at four o'clock.'

Holding the face beside the witchdoctor's eye, I pointed to the place where the hour hand would be at four o'clock.'

Daudi peered into the witchdoctor's eye, carefully inspecting the corresponding spot.

'*Heehee*,' he nodded, 'I see it, Bwana, a thing small as the dust.'

'*Hongo*,' said Ng'oma, 'it is large as a brick to me. It grinds its way into my head.'

Straightening myself, I selected instruments from the makeshift steriliser poised over a primus stove.

'We will use this special one, Daudi. It is called a *spud*, I said in English.

'Oh,' replied Daudi in the same tongue, 'but is not a spud a potato?'

Smiling, I explained. Then taking up a position behind Ng'oma, I rested his head against my shirt and told him to look up. He did so but his eyes rolled wildly.

'Do not make your eye move round and round like a mad dog,' I ordered. 'Keep it still and look at my nose.'

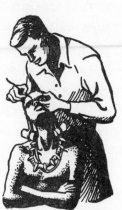

'*Yoh*,' he said thickly, 'but why, Bwana?'

'It is a very useful nose,' I replied, smiling.

'But what is the purpose?' he persisted.

For a moment his eye was quiet. The spud touched the deeply embedded bit of grit, the eye suddenly blinked and my chance was gone.

'*Hee*,' said Ng'oma again, 'what is the purpose?'

'Of noses?' I asked, smiling.

'No, Bwana, of looking at them.'

'It gives you something large to rest your eye on, so that it may not move.'

He concentrated and the eye was still.

'*Twi*, Ng'oma! Keep it still – not a move – that's it – quietly – there is no pain – no move – ooh!'

'*Kah*, Bwana,' Ng'oma's voice was very apologetic. 'I tried with strength, the eye, however, insisted.' He blinked rapidly.

'*Kumbe*,' said Daudi, 'rest a while and the Bwana will attack again.'

I adjusted the head mirror. The speck in the witchdoctor's eye hardly looked worth worrying about but I knew the searing pain and the great danger to sight that was present if it were not removed and its minute resting-place thoroughly cleaned.

'No blinking now,' I ordered.

A hush fell on the ward. With eyes fixed on that tiny black spot in his dark brown eye, I directed the point of the spud. It grated against the grit which moved. I gave the instrument the slightest upward pressure and the foreign body was out.

'Gone,' I grunted. The word was echoed round the ward.

'Morfe *fluorescin*, the green medicine,' I ordered.

Daudi complied and a deep green patch appeared where the grit had torn a minute hole. With a sharpened match-stick dipped in carbolic I cauterized this, carefully touching every damaged spot.

'Bwana, why do that?' asked Ng'oma.

'There must be no *dudu*, no germ, remaining in your eye ulcer. My small stick is doing in miniature the same thing as when you put a glowing stick from the fire on to a scorpion in a hole.'

There was a nodding of heads, *'heheeh!'*

Old Ng'wagu lay back in his bed and spoke softly to no one in particular:

'Kumbe, the Bwana has strong medicine and much wisdom in the matter of eyes. Do not even the witchdoctors acknowledge this?'

11
The Block

By the light of a hurricane-lantern a junior dispenser was busily engaged in removing all Ng'wagu's hair, using a gigantic pair of scissors.

'*Kumbe*,' said the old man, 'truly I have arrived. Will the Bwana work soon on my eyes?'

'*Bado*, soon, but not yet,' replied the dispenser, clipping away vigorously.

Another dispenser with a large smile on his face was carrying a watering-can full of water. This would be Ng'wagu's bath. The drums in the village were going by the time the old man was put to bed. A palm-leaf mat was the only 'kapok' mattress that separated him from the wire mattress of the stretcher. His bedding consisted of two unbleached calico sheets and a cotton blanket. The pillow, also made from unbleached calico, was stuffed with grass. The old minstrel, Ng'wagu, yawned and stretched himself.

'*Yah*,' he said, 'this is the place for sleep.' He was silent for quite a while and then he moved and grunted. '*Heh,* but behold, this bed bites a little.'

Daudi chuckled. 'It takes a little while to get used to that wire beneath you, but you do in time. Although, behold, in the morning you have a pattern upon your back.'

'*Hongo*, Bwana.' Ng'wagu raised his voice to attract my attention. 'I would taste the medicine of the hospital.'

I nodded and a large dose of green medicine was given. I well knew it had an awful taste, but the old man smacked his lips. '*Yoh*,' he said, settling down to sleep, 'that's medicine.'

Next morning, if Ng'wagu had been able to see, he would have been convinced that it had been the bed that bit him, and the bed only, for Daudi and his team of dispensers were very busy with a painter's blow lamp, petrol tins full of very hot water and pyrethrum powder mixed in kerosene. Any stray flora or fauna or, if you prefer the African word, *dudus*, that found their way into that hospital with visitors were given a very hot reception, every Thursday morning.

Ng'wagu was sitting in the sun with his sheet over his head. He was obviously feeling in good form. Round him was grouped a series of other patients and the old man, sitting with his back to the whitewashed wall, sang with vigour. The thing that intrigued me was the way his big toes moved, keeping time with his singing. As he came to the end of a verse the whole staff joined in the chorus. The concert was curtailed by the arrival of the eye-dresser.

'Great One,' he said, 'your bed is ready for you again. Come in. Preparations must be made for your operation.'

Quite an elaborate training was given to all patients who were to have the cataract removed from their eyes. Kefa stood behind the end of his bed.

'Great One, this is what will happen on the day that the Bwana removes the *cipece*, the cataract, from your eye. Those who obey the Bwana without any wobble – they are the ones whose eyes see the most. *Hongo*, but those who do not obey very completely, *huh*, their lot is one of trouble and sadness, and perhaps of continued darkness.'

'*Kumbe*,' said the old man, 'show me what I should do.'

'*Heh*,' said Kefa, 'lie still on your back. Look down, down at your feet. No, *down! Down!* Yes, there!' He pushed the old man's chin. 'That's down, *down!*'

Ng'wagu rolled his eyes and looked anywhere but down.

'*Heh*,' said Kefa, looking at me with a smile on his face but his voice very firm. 'You must not make your eyes go round and round like the *ibis* bird in the days of the locusts. They must be still, *twi*, absolutely quiet.'

For some ten minutes Kefa kept up his instructions until the old man knew where his eyes were actually directed. Then drops were put in. He did it very gently, but as the drop went into his eye, the old man rose a good three inches off the bed, his eyelids closed almost with a snap, as did his mouth.

'*Yah*,' he said, '*yah*, what was that?'

'*Kah*,' said the smiling dispenser, 'it was just a drop of medicine put into your eye. *Kah*, if you jump like that there will be trouble. Great One, you must learn to relax.'

There was an interested group of spectators watching all that was happening, and then came Daudi with a pair of scissors. He snipped a charm from round the old man's midriff, another charm that was round his neck. He put them in an envelope.

'Great One,' he said, 'this is a place of wisdom, not a place of charms. We will help you, but behold, the charms have gone. We have the better way.'

I could see Ng'oma, the witchdoctor, looking over the heads of some of the other patients, his mouth wide open. Then Daudi picked up a sheet of glass from the table.

'*Hongo*, I will explain to you that this blindness, this darkness that causes you sorrow is not due to anger of the ancestors. It is not due to spirits who wish you evil. This is the cause, and this is the answer. Watch.' He held the glass up. 'Great Ones, can you see through this?' There was a nodding of heads as he held it a few inches above his face. He wiped it with the sleeve of his shirt. 'Behold there is no dirt upon this glass, and therefore you can see through it.' Again there came the nodding of heads.

Old Ng'wagu said, 'Tell me, what are you doing?'

As this was being explained to him, Daudi went outside to where the camp fire had burned last night. He took some of the ashes and mixed them with a few drops of water. Coming back, he held this mixture in his hand and gave the glass to Kefa. Taking the white paste, he rubbed it over the glass and again he held it between himself and Ng'oma, the witchdoctor.

'Great One, can you see my face now?'

'*Ng'o, Ng'o*,' said Ng'oma, shaking his head. 'Behold the ashes on the glass make it white. You cannot see through it.'

Kefa slowly drew aside the glass. There was nothing between Ng'oma's eyes and Daudi's face.

'Great One,' said Daudi, 'can you see my face now?'

'*Heh*,' Ng'oma nodded, 'there is nothing in the way.'

Daudi nodded. 'Behold, in the eye, does not the same thing happen? For you, and for me, O Ng'oma, within our eye is a thing like this glass which helps us to see clearly, but should it get smeared with disease, then it becomes like the glass. You cannot see through it. Remove it and you can see again.'

'*Kah*,' said Ng'oma, 'it is a work of great difficulty, to remove from within a man's eye the trouble that is there.'

'*Hongo*, but it is the work of the Bwana to do that. He has skill in these things'... he laid his hand on Ng'wagu's shoulder... 'if the one upon whom he works does exactly what he is told.'

'*Kumbe*,' said the old man, 'these things will I do if you will show me how. But will it not hurt me?'

'*Heh*,' said Daudi, ' a little, but only a little. But when you lie in bed for four days with your eyes bandaged, and you are very quiet, and you do not cough, you do not move, you do only the smallest movements, then, behold, there is comfort.'

'*Kah*, it is a small thing if I get my eyes to see again.'

'As you lie there, Great One, think of the Son of God who is the light, not only of your eye, but who brings light to your soul, who takes away the dark thing that stops the light coming in, that you may see God. As you cannot remove the block from within your eye, so you cannot remove the block of sin from within your soul. That is the work of the Great Doctor, Jesus Himself.'

As Daudi spoke I was looking through the window, thinking how much more effective it was that Africans should tell the story of the Good News of light coming into darkness, rather than that the doctor who operated should be the only one to speak. Suddenly I was aware of another peculiar cavalcade of people coming down towards the hospital gates. First came a tall youth with red mud in his hair dressed in slightly less than the minimum of clothing. Behind him came an old man, walking on the heel of one foot and the

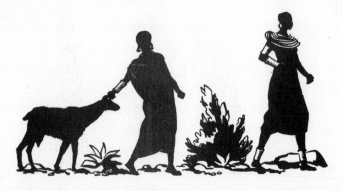

toes of the other, a knobbed stick in the right hand while in the left he clasped another stick which was in the hands of a small boy ahead of him who gently led him along the smoothest portion of the track. Behind them came three women: one had a basket of flour on her head, the second had no food, while the third was dragging along a rather pungent goat.

They walked through the gate of the hospital and out of my view. A minute or two later Daudi arrived at the door.

'Bwana, an old man has come who has cataract trouble. *Heh*, he is one of independence. He would not have the help of his family. His feet are hurt, his ear is injured, and, Bwana, he is full of words, words of grumbling.'

'Right,' I said, 'I'll see him and do what I can for him,' but little did I realise how much trouble had walked into our hospital that morning.

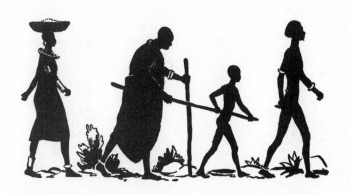

12

Meeting a Grumbler

'*Yayagwe, yayagwe,*' said my newest patient sitting on the three-legged stool in our out-patient room. '*Kumbe*, Bwana, my troubles are great.'

Daudi behind me whispered, 'Bwana, truly do they call him *Muzozi*, the noisy one, while there are some who call him *Ng'ung'uliko*, the grumbler.'

'*Heh, heh*, Daudi, he sounds like both mixed up altogether.'

The old man started speaking again. 'Bwana, I have been in trouble. Behold, did I not walk one night into the fire?'

'*Kah*,' said one of his relations, '*kah*, did we not tell you we had moved the fireplace? Did we not tell you to tell us when you wanted to go inside the door?'

'*Kah*,' shouted the old man, 'shall I not do my own things? Shall I not walk by myself?'

'*Mbeka,* truly,' interrupted one of his relations, 'will you not walk down holes and bruise your legs?'

Ng'ung'uliko caressed his shin-bones as the voice went on, 'And will you not walk into thorn trees and destroy your ears as you have done?'

My latest patient's hand unconsciously went towards his ear lobes which had been stretched so that each would easily have held a tennis ball. One was intact but the other was torn and draggled forlornly down almost to his shoulder. The grumbler raised his voice to such a pitch that it was impossible for anyone else to speak.

'*Yah,*' he whined, 'I'm a miserable man. My feet ache, my bones ache, my body is bruised, my ear gives me sorrow.'

'Courage, Great One of the tribe,' I answered. 'I'll fix you up. We'll give you medicine for your pain. We'll paint other medicines over your burns and make them better. They'll all heal in time.'

'*Kumbe,*' he said, 'but what about my ears, Bwana, my beautiful ears? They were my pride, Bwana, but now … *yayagwe!*' He shook his head dolefully.

Daudi grinned across at me, as we watched him pick up tenderly the two ends of his ear lobes. 'Behold, Bwana, this was once my pride and delight, and now, *kah*, it is just two bits of meat.' He lapsed into a series of unintelligible grunts and groans.

Daudi started applying dressings to the old man's burnt feet. I could hear his high-pitched grumblings as he was transferred to the ward, as his hair was cut, '*yayagwe,*' as he was bathed, '*yayagwe.*' From the bathroom came his voice, full of complaint, 'I refuse completely.' Then came a gurgle and Daudi's voice, very kind but very firm.

Late that afternoon Kefa was putting Ng'wagu and Ng'ung'uliko, the grumbler, through their paces. 'Look down,' he said, 'down.'

Ng'wagu had mastered this technique and his eyes slowly moved down and looked sightlessly at his feet, but the grumbler rolled his eyes. 'Why should I look down,' he said, 'when I want to look up? Why should I?'

'Because,' said Kefa patiently, 'the Bwana would move the trouble from your eye, therefore look down at your feet, down.'

'*Kah, kah*, I do not have comfort in looking down.'

Kefa moved over to Ng'wagu's bed. 'The second thing you must learn is to look with your left eye towards your nose, your nose.'

The old man moved his eye slowly in the right direction.

'*Heh*,' said Kefa, 'that's good. That's good. Now always remember that you must not move suddenly when the Bwana is working on your eyes, no matter how much noise there is.'

He dropped a kerosene tin. '*Kaaaaaah!*' said Ng'ung'uliko, jumping a good foot into the air. '*Kah*, what was that?'

Ng'wagu was on his elbow. 'What, why, how?'

'*Yah*,' said Kefa, 'you must lie still no matter what noises happen. It might be that something is spilt and if you move quickly your eyes will be ruined.'

113

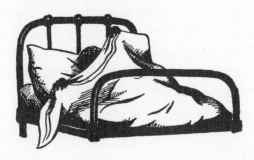

'*Kah, kah*, this is a thing of great sorrow. What shall I do? *Yayagwe*, oh, my mother!'

The grumbler pulled the blankets over his head and continued his lamentations underneath it. Drops were put carefully into Ng'wagu's eyes. This time there was no movement. '*Hongo*,' he said, 'they do not hurt. They make my eyes feel there is less sandiness in them.'

'*Heh*,' nodded Kefa, 'that is right. That is how it should be. Have comfort, Great One, the Bwana will help before many days are past. These are the days of preparation. Must we not prepare the soil before the seed is planted?'

Next morning Daudi was dressing the grumbler's feet.

'*Hongo*,' I said, 'Great One, do not your feet feel comfortable today?'

'*Heh, heh*,' said the old man, 'Bwana, there is less pain there, but oh, I have pains in my *cigongo*, my back. The bed bites me.'

'Be thankful,' said Daudi, 'that it is nothing worse. The teeth of *ikutupa*, the tick, are less kindly. The small, sharp nose of *izuguni*, the mosquito, brings sorrow.' He went on with a collection of the not-so-nice activities of less social insects.

Kefa wanted to show me what Ng'wagu could do. 'Bwana, watch.' He turned to his patient. 'Look down, Great One.' The old man looked down. 'Look towards your nose.' His eyes moved in that direction. 'Look towards your ear, your northern ear.'

Before Ng'wagu could comply with this order, the blind man in the next bed let out a wail, 'Oh, Bwana, what of my ear, my beautiful ear? Behold, there is no joy in it. Once it was my pride.'

Kefa rolled his eyes. We were a little tired of Ng'ung'uliko's pride in his ears.

'When your feet have recovered a little, then I will take you on safari to the room where we mend people and on that day I will return your ear to what it used to be.'

'*Hongo*,' said the old man grasping my hand. 'Bwana, do not deceive me. Do not tell me lies. Oh, *yah*.'

Ng'wagu from the next bed put his hand out towards me. 'Bwana,' he said. I bent over him. 'Behold, I hope the grumbler does not upset you greatly. He is full of words.

'*Hongo*, Bwana, I can understand how he feels. You cannot know what it feels like to have been blind for years and years. To feel that your children think of you only as a useless one. Bwana, the rain falls and you know that you cannot dig in the garden. You hear the others laughing and playing their games, but, *yah*, you're in darkness.' He let out a sigh. 'There is no joy in living in darkness.'

'Truly, my friend, for that reason Jesus said, "I am the Light of the World." When He comes, darkness

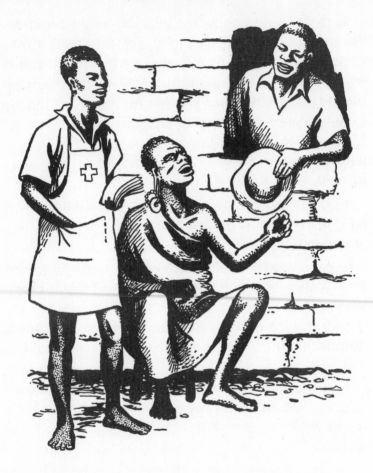

just disappears. You find the way to walk. There can be no darkness where He is, for He takes sin away and sin always brings darkness, and as you know, with darkness comes sadness and misery.'

The grumbler was sitting up in bed. Almost in a scream he said, '*Zinghani na zinghani na zinghani!* Words, words!' He was almost frantic.

At that moment Ng'wagu was shuffling to his feet. 'Bwana, I would go into the sun where I may talk with the old men.'

'*Hongo*,' I said, 'a good idea. There you may sing the words that will bring comfort to your mind and joy to the ears of all but Ng'ung'uliko.'

As Ng'wagu sat down on the stool that the dispenser provided for him, the round, smiling face of Tadayo, the singer, appeared at the dispensary window.

'*Yah*,' he said, '*kah*, it is the old one. We will sing for him. He, too, shall sing for us. *Heh,* he has the voice of strength.'

Tadayo removed his battered hat and started to sing. As the chorus came along, old Ng'wagu threw his head back and sang with the dispensers and the others round the place, but as the sound died away, from within the ward came a disgruntled voice.

'Words, words, words! I will have nothing to with this thing you talk about. *Heh*, mine is a life of sadness. *Heh*, my feet, my ears, my eyes.'

13

Eyewitness

Old Ng'ung'uliko sat up in his bed looking much more cheerful than usual. He put out his hand and gripped mine.

'*Kah*, Bwana, behold you are my father and my mother.'

'Here, wait a minute,' I interrupted, 'I don't see that.'

Daudi grinned broadly as the old African voice went on.

'*Heh*, you have taken the pain from my feet, the bruises give me no sorrow, and…'

'*Kah*,' said Daudi, 'the bed no longer bites.'

You could hear the smile in his voice, but this goaded the grumbler almost into a frenzy.

'*Yah*,' he wailed, 'but my ears, my beautiful ears. *Heh*, you have mended my feet, and soothed my burns and bumps, but nothing can ever mend my ears.'

'*Wacho*, Great One, *heh*, don't you believe a word of it. This is a work of small difficulty, this matter of ears.'

Again the old man got up on his elbow, gripping my arm. 'But how, Bwana, won't it hurt? When will you do it? How will you do it?'

'Hold hard, Great One, one question at a time. First, it won't hurt. I will squirt medicine into your ears that will stop all pain. When? I'll do it today before sundown. How? With my special weapon, in the room where we operate. Now are you happy?'

'*Lunji*, perhaps, but Bwana, I shall want my son to stand and watch and tell me if the work is done properly.'

'*Viswanu*, all right, but he must follow out the custom of our hospital. If he promises to do this he may watch.'

So it was arranged. At four o'clock in the afternoon I walked to the theatre. There was quite an amazing scene at the door. Ng'ung'uliko's son very unwillingly was being sprayed with insecticide, enthusiastically, by Daudi, who then fitted him out with a mask and a gown, led him into the theatre and placed him behind a cupboard. As I scrubbed my hands for the

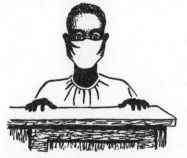

operation I could see his eyes peering ludicrously over the top of the white mask, the square of white gauze accentuating the blackness of his face.

'Don't you move,' Daudi frowned ominously. 'Stay as you are, where you are.'

'*Kumbe*, I will follow your words,' said the head, who obviously was deeply impressed by the whole proceedings.

The old man was carried in on a stretcher and placed on the operating table.

'To help ears, the mouth must be shut,' I ordered.

Towels were placed in position. Daudi carefully washed the ear with soap and water, using a gauze swab. Then I painted the area with iodine and injected local anaesthetic. The scene is set for the operation. The old man lies on the table. At his feet, facing us, half hidden by a cupboard, his son peers at us. I am standing on the right side of the table. On the palm of my hand lie two ends of ear lobe, about half the thickness of a lead pencil. Into each of these an injection has been made, right up close where they joined the ears. From underneath the piece of gauze that covers his face comes from Ng'ung'uliko a series of groans and grumbles. Before the operation actually takes place, we pray and ask God for help, and then I snip a quarter of an inch from each of the trailing ear lobes.

'*Yoh*,' gasped the son, obviously on tiptoe behind his mask. '*Heh!*'

'*Nhawule*, what's the matter?' asked the patient.

'Did that hurt you, father?'

'Did what hurt?'

'*Kumbe*, the Bwana cut you with his scissors.'

'*Kah*, he did nothing of the sort.'

'*Heh*, I did,' I laughed as I stitched up the cut ends, reuniting the lobe, 'and what is more, I have nearly finished sewing your ear up. It is nearly repaired.'

'*Kah*,' said the old man, '*yah*, who'd have believed it? Has he truly done it, my son?'

'*Eeh*,' nodded the son, 'but I don't think that your ears are both the same size now. Did not the Bwana remove a little bit?'

Ng'ung'uliko struggled to rise, the gauze billowing up and down as he stuttered in rage.

'*Yah*, behold, I knew there was deception in it. *Heh*, my ears were the most beautiful in the village. They were both the same size, and now…' His voice trailed off into a whine. He shook his head. '*Heh, kumbe*, truly I am miserable.'

'Cheer up, Great One,' I laughed, 'the operation isn't finished yet. Your ears will be exactly the same size. Behold, am I not going to take a tuck in the other side?'

Ng'ung'uliko muttered again and again, 'a tuck, a tuck.'

His son's eyes seemed to protrude still further. Daudi was chuckling away to himself as I carefully measured the two ear lobes, and repeated the surgical procedure, and measured again. The lobes were the same size to the fraction of an inch.

I put down the scissors. 'There, Great One, the work is finished. They are the same size exactly, and in a month's time you will be able to put all your ornaments back into them.'

His hand reached out for mine from underneath the blankets.

'*Yah*, Bwana, truly this is a thing of amazement. *Yah*, behold, it has never been done before in all our country.'

He sang my praises solidly for twenty-four hours, urging patients and visitors to 'see the wisdom of the Bwana.'

I thought we had cured his grumbling for life, but three days later, as I did the rounds in the ward, I heard him at it again.

'*Yayagwe*, oh my mother,' he lamented, 'my feet are repaired truly. My ears are renewed, but behold, it is a work of no profit, for I will only walk into another fire and burn my feet again, and again tear my ears.'

'Have patience, O chief of grumblers,' I laughed.

The pitch of the old man's voice rose. 'You haven't removed the cause of my trouble, Bwana. I am blind. I've lived in darkness for ten years.'

'*Hongo*, then follow my words carefully, and let me give you back your eyesight.'

The old man almost hissed the words at me. 'Do not jest with me. *Kah!* There are none who can see when they've been blind for years as I have.'

'Your words are false. The Bwana is able to give sight back. *Heh*, did he not do it for me?'

A score of eyes turned to the doorway where stood an elderly man, a chief, Mesomapya by name.

'*Hongo*, have I not come to greet the Bwana? My gift is without.' He pointed through the door with his chin. I could see a woman with a basket on her head containing eggs.

The Chief went on, 'I lay in this bed.' His hand touched the pillow. 'They told me to look up, to look down, to look towards my northern ear.'

I noticed that as he spoke Ng'wagu laboriously followed out instructions, his eyes following the directions that the Chief gave. Ng'ung'uliko was on one elbow, drinking in the whole story avidly.

'Truly,' went on the Chief, 'I did exactly what I was told. Where I was told to look, I looked. No noise upset me.'

At that moment Kefa dropped a dish, making an appalling crash. The grumbler leapt half out of bed, muttering with a mixture of fear and indignation. Ng'wagu had a slow smile on his face.

'*Heh*,' he chuckled, 'see, I was not upset by noise. Did I not lie still?'

Mesomapya went on. 'The Bwana did his work of cutting. *Cipece*, the cataract, was removed, and now I see. I walk in light. *Kumbe*, but only because I followed the words of the Bwana.'

'*Hongo*, that is the path I, too, shall follow,' said Ng'wagu, swinging his legs over the side of the bed. 'I shall look down, at the word of the Bwana. I shall not move unless the Bwana allows me to. Noises shall not disturb me. Even if Simba, the lion, roars…'

'What then, Great One?'

'*Heh*, I shall lie quiet.'

'But should Daudi sing, what then?'

'*Kah*,' said the old man, 'I, too, should sing, like this …'

He gripped his stick and his eyes peered sightlessly ahead. For a moment his head moved to and fro as though he were trying to catch the rhythm and then he burst into song. He was still singing as Daudi and I walked down to the operating theatre to make sure that our cataract knives were ready for the operation in two or three days' time.

Daudi was carrying the microscope. We moved the operating table over to the window. He placed the microscope on it and brought out the narrow-bladed cataract knives. One by one I put them underneath the lens, after juggling with the mirror and focusing. I looked at the first and held it up.

'What do you think of that, Daudi?'

'It looks all right, Bwana, but we had trouble with it, you remember.'

'*Heh*, just look here then and you'll see why.' My African helper skilfully adjusted the instrument and whistled softly.

'*Heh*, Bwana, it looks like a saw. I'll pack it with the others. They'll have to be sent to London for sharpening.'

'I'm going to talk about that knife tomorrow at prayers, Daudi. It looks all right, but it doesn't cut. And when you see it under the mike, well, it's obvious what's wrong.'

Daudi nodded. 'I see, Bwana. We may look quite ordinary in the eyes of people. We may be just as good as the other knives in the box, comparatively, but what matters is that neither we nor they have any value in getting on with the job.'

'*Heh*, Daudi, and only the searching eye of Almighty God picks out the trouble and only He can repair it.'

'*Kumbe*, Bwana, does it not underline what Jesus said, "I am the Way and the Truth and the Life. No one comes to the Father except through me"?'

'Truly, Daudi, there's only one way, but it's amazing how people try to side-step.'

I took up the second knife and after careful examination discarded it too. Daudi handed me a third.

'Now, look at that. It's a beauty.'

There wasn't a blemish in the instrument. It was true right through.

'Now, that's the one we'll use for both Ng'ung'uliko and Ng'wagu. They ought to be ready for the operation before the week is out.'

14
Training

'If we go the ordinary way about training Ng'ung'uliko, Bwana,' said Kefa, 'we will have no chance whatsoever of operating on his eyes. Behold, he performs with small wisdom. Tell him to look up and he looks down. Tell him to look at his nose and he looks at everything but that. *Yah*, we must try other ways of preparing him.'

'*Heh*, well what do you suggest?'

'Bwana, let us tell him that he is one who has less strength of will than his companion, Ng'wagu, who when told to look at his feet, looks in that direction. Let us just use a little scorn and see if that is the right medicine.'

An hour or two later, as I sat writing up the record book in the men's ward, I saw Kefa talking to Daudi.

'*Heh*,' said Kefa in a voice you could hear all over the place. 'It is a pity that Ng'ung'uliko here has not the wisdom of his companion. Behold, you tell Ng'wagu to look at his feet, and *yah*, his eyes are in that direction in very fast time. *Heh*, but Ng'ung'uliko, it is a pity. He is an old man. He has had many troubles. It is perhaps not his own fault. He cannot do these things. Behold…'

An enraged voice came from the bed: 'Who cannot look at his feet if he wants to? Who cannot look at his nose if he wants to? *Heh*, behold, my eyes may have small power, but *yah*, I can do what I wish.'

'*Hoh*,' said Kefa, 'then look at your feet.'

Ng'ung'uliko's eyes moved in that direction and stayed there.

'Look at your nose.'

His eyes went in the right direction.

'Look up.'

He did it without a quiver, without a murmur.

'*Yah*,' said Kefa, 'behold, he is a man of great courage and tremendous will-power.'

There was a grin on Daudi's face.

Ng'ung'uliko snapped back. 'Of course I am.'

'*Heheh*, we will speak to the Bwana, and it may be tomorrow we can operate.'

I got up from the table and went across, first to Ng'wagu, and pulled down his eyelids. The eyes looked in good form. You cannot operate if there are any signs of infection.

The old man whispered to me, 'Bwana, will it be tomorrow? Can you do the work then?'

'*Heh*, if all goes well, and it seems to be going well, tomorrow is the day.'

Said the old man, 'That will be joy, Bwana, that will be joy.'

I pulled down Ng'ung'uliko's eyelids. There wasn't a quiver or a complaint.

'*Hongo*,' I said, 'the eye looks well. Behold, tomorrow will be your day as well. Today, Kefa, the eyes must be washed very thoroughly, many drops put in, much preparation. But first I must test out these men. Behold, I will see who obeys best, and he shall be the first to be operated on.'

I stood at the end of the bed and gave orders to those two old men, as keen to obey as any soldier on a parade ground.

'Look up.' Their eyes moved slowly up and stayed still.

'Look north.' Their eyes moved in that direction.

'Back to normal.' They came back and stayed still.

I nodded to Daudi who upset a stool and made a tremendous clatter. There wasn't so much as the closing of an eyelid from either of them.

'Good,' I said, 'splendid, that's the thing. Now, Ng'wagu, what would you do in the operation if suddenly you felt a large ant climbing up your leg?'

'Bwana,' said the old man, 'I would tell you and keep very still.'

'*Heh*, that is right. Ng'ung'uliko, what you do if you suddenly felt that you wanted to cough?'

'Bwana, I should stop myself from coughing and tell you.'

'That's right. Now don't forget these things, men. Now look down.'

Both of them looked down carefully. I patted them both on the shoulders.

'That's the thing. Do that tomorrow and with the good hand of God upon mine light will come back to you, *if* you obey my instructions, not only during the operation but in the days that are to follow. You must lie absolutely still on these beds. You must under no circumstances touch the bandages that will be over your eyes. If you want anything, tell us. We will help. Do you understand fully?'

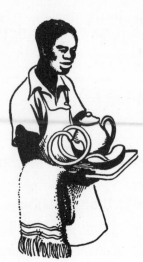

They nodded and I felt that the whole thing was firmly in their memories.

Kefa had returned to the wards with a most amusing apparatus. It consisted of a large teapot with a rubber tube over the broken spout. The rubber tube ended in a minute glass affair which was used to wash out the eye. Kefa held what is called a kidney bowl, shaped to fit in with the contour of the face, underneath Ng'wagu's eyes and proceeded to wash them out very carefully. Drops were put in. Everything was in order for the next day's big job.

'Give each of them a little pill,' I ordered. 'Behold, when night comes let them sleep, for tomorrow may be a day of difficulties. They must have sleep and rest beforehand.'

But tomorrow's difficulties weren't what I expected them to be. In the early morning I made my final inspection of eyes. Ng'ung'uliko's eyes were looking very well. There was no sign of redness or inflammation. The eyelids were clean. There was no sign of any sore or anything that would block me from operating. He seemed surprisingly cheerful and told me that he had slept well. I went across to the next bed and pulled the eyelid down. Daudi's voice over my shoulder said:

'*Kah*, how could that have happened, Bwana?'

The eyes were red and ugly-looking.

'*Yah*, Ng'wagu.'

'What's the trouble, Bwana?'

'Behold, there are *dudus* – germs – that have got into your eyes. They are red. It would be unsafe for us to work upon your eyes today. If we did they would never be better.'

The old minstrel's face dropped, disappointment was written on every feature.

'*Yah*,' he said, 'Bwana, I have done all that you told me to do.'

'Have comfort. I have medicine which will kill these *dudus*. It is only a matter of a few more days in bed, and *yah*…'

'*Yah*,' said the old man. 'Bwana, it means darkness is still upon me and light is further away.'

Even as he spoke, I put the appropriate drugs into his eyes.

'More courage, Great One. Already the *dudus* are having sorrow for the medicine that I have put in. Before many days have gone your sight will be back with you again.'

'But, Bwana, can't you operate today?'

'*Ng'o*, not today.'

He let out a gusty sigh and then, softly to himself, hummed over his favourite tune. I bent down so that only he and I could hear.

'Behold, Great One, when God lets things like this happen, He has a reason. I have found this many times, and behold, perhaps in a week's time you and I will know the reason why today your eyes are not fit to work on. In these things it is important that we should leave ourselves in His hands. Sometimes, if we had the choice, we would go ahead fast, and He blocks us. Many times this has happened to me and always there has been a reason. '

The old man nodded his head. 'Bwana, I am beginning to understand these things. Surely the help of God is ours.' He raised his voice, and when Ng'ung'uliko in the next bed heard the words 'help of God,' he said:

'*Kah*, I am strong enough myself to do what I wish to do. Behold, when the Bwana operates today, I will do the things that he says. *Heh*.'

A spate of words followed this.

It was late in the afternoon when the operating theatre was set up, and he was carried down on a stretcher. Once again his son was masked and gowned and stood behind the cupboard, watching what was being done. Once again the old man lay on the table and it would have been difficult to have found a more cooperative patient. The eye bandage was carefully put on and Ng'ung'uliko went back to the ward, clutching between his thumb and finger a piece of cotton wool and holding the cataract which was about the size of a split pea.

'Great One,' I said, 'you have behaved with great courage. Now for four days you must lie still, very still, and above all things you must not touch that bandage over your eyes.'

'*Heh*,' said the old man, nodding.

But as Daudi and I watched him being carried through the door, the dispenser shook his head.

'Bwana, I have fears for that one. He will not obey.'

'Truly, Daudi, the operation was a great success. Seldom have we had a better one, but behold there are many links in that chain and if one of them breaks down then the whole thing falls.'

'*Kumbe*, Bwana. What I feel is that he will rub his eyes at night because they're itchy. *Heh*, I am afraid that he will follow the wrong way.'

'*Kah*, isn't that the same thing that crops up in the disease of our soul? We obey in many things, but Jesus says if we disobey, or offend in one point, we are guilty of the whole thing. Of course, God could make us obey. He could paralyse the tongue just as you were about to tell a lie, or to make mangoes disappear from the tree when you felt like stealing them.'

'*Kah*, Bwana,' laughed Daudi, 'wouldn't the world be a mad place if that sort of thing happened? Wouldn't people complain?'

'*Kumbe*, what about the idea of tying the grumbler's hands to the side of the bed so that he cannot rub his eyes?'

'*Heh*, Bwana, he has been called the grumbler and the noisy one. Do that and you will see what he does. *Yah*.'

15

Set-back

'*Chai*, Bwana,' said Kefa bringing a tray into my office.

'*Chai* of *saa kumi*, the tenth hour,' (or if you prefer it, in the English way of telling time, four in the afternoon) 'and, Bwana, as you drink, think that today is the third day and Ng'ung'uliko has not grumbled. He has not even complained that the bed has bitten him. Bwana, this is a thing of wonder.' Kefa smiled. 'Tomorrow, Bwana, the bandages will come off, and *yah*, will he have joy if he sees again!'

'*When* he sees again,' retorted Daudi. 'There was never a better operation than the one that the Bwana did on him. *Heh*, everything went splendidly.'

The sun set and I was still in that office trying to balance the hospital accounts. After my evening meal of tough Tanganyikan chicken, spinach and sweet potato, I went back to my office armed with a hurricane-lantern. As I went through the door I could hear the singing of the folk round the camp fire.

I opened the window and looked out on the scene. Ng'wagu was sitting there singing very heartily indeed. On each side of him were two old men whom I recognised as recent cataract cases, both of whom had been good results.

One of these old men said, '*Kumbe*, the Bwana has pills to make eyes better. Behold, there are very many of our tribe whom he has helped.'

'*Heh*,' said the second man, 'he certainly helped me, but behold, I should not like to have been the first one upon whom he did this work.'

'*Hongo*,' came Daudi's voice, 'I will tell you that story. When the Bwana lived amongst his relations in the country where the skin of people is white, he went along to the place where meat is sold, and said to the one who sells meat, "I would buy the eyes of pigs that I may work upon them."'

'*Heh*,' said the old man, 'did they not think this was witchcraft that the Bwana was doing?'

'*Heh*, they did not think that at all, but they wondered what the Bwana would do. *Heh*, he took the pigs' eyes to his house and put them in a lump of clay mixed with oil, and worked upon them with his little knife as he worked upon your eye. At first he worked with small skill, and then as he did many of them, behold, it was work without great difficulty, and then the Bwana came here to Tanganyika. Behold, we used the room over there.' He pointed with his chin to a whitewashed building. 'It was in that room that the Bwana first worked upon an eye that was in a man's head. First he talked with me many words, and told me all about it. He showed me what to do that I might help. We practised the work together many times without anybody being there and then we practised it with someone being there and the Bwana used no knife, only a little piece of cotton wool, so that all the actions might be understood. One day he did the operation.

'*Heh*, the Bwana had little calmness. He looked this way and that. He had no joy in the voice of the crows. Did he not say, "*Yoh*, stone the crows?" And when I asked him if he could feel his heart bumping against his ribs, he smiled and said, "*Heeh*, Daudi, it would be wise if we filled some bags with sand that I might rest my elbow upon it, for behold, see my hand shakes. This is a bad thing."

'And then the time came. The blind man lay on the table in that room. The Bwana put drops into his eyes and I feared as I saw the way that the eye-dropper quivered. We prayed with words before the Bwana started, and then, all of us prayed very strongly with our thoughts as he worked. The Bwana rested his elbow on the sandbag. He told the old man to look down. I could see his teeth set. *Heh*, behold, *nghuguti,* sweat, ran down his forehead. But, *kumbe*, the hand of Almighty God was upon the Bwana's, for the operation, though very slow, was most successful. *Kumbe*, I do not know who had the greater joy, the Bwana, or the blind man, when the bandages were take off. It was a time of great interest. This is what happened.

'"Behold, I can see," said our patient.

'The Bwana gripped him by the shoulder and said, "Really, can you truly?"'

'*Heh*,' laughed the folk around the fire. '*Heh,* it was a thing of joy.'

'*Kumbe*, and how we listened,' went on Daudi, 'as the Bwana told him that you could not get rid of blindness by what you did yourself, but you had to have the right help from outside. He showed the old man his *cipece*, his cataract, and told him it was like sin, that it blocked the light from coming in and that only Jesus could take away the other cataract from a man's heart, a trouble much greater than anything in man's eye. *Hongo*, I have heard this hundreds of times, but every time I understand more clearly what sin is like and how it works to produce soul-blindness, how it makes you miserable, how when you walk in darkness you can only come to trouble.'

'*Kumbe*,' said Ng'wagu, 'should I not know that better than you? Do I not walk in darkness now?'

'*Heh*,' said the old men beside him, 'we walked in darkness, but now we walk in light. Behold, the Bwana preaches a very strong sermon with his little knife. How can you forget these things when light is back in your eye?'

'These are words of joy,' laughed Ng'wagu. 'We will sing.' And sing they did.

Back in the office, I added up the last column of figures, the books balanced. I closed them with a sigh, and felt how very worthwhile it was to be a Jungle Doctor. I looked up at the picture on the wall, Holman Hunt's "Light of the World," and I prayed that God would allow me the chance of helping many other people to understand about the "Light of the World."

Suddenly an urgent voice came from within the ward.

'Where is the Bwana? Quickly!'

'*Heh*,' said Daudi, 'his light is still on in the office.'

I heard flying footsteps and Kefa was at the door.

'Bwana,' he gasped, '*tabu sana*, great trouble! It's Ng'ung'uliko. *Heh*, he has pulled the bandage off, he has gone back to the ways of *muganga*, the witchdoctor. He has put saliva in his eyes, and, Bwana, he is making great trouble.'

I grabbed the lantern and hurried after the African dispenser. Sure enough, the eye bandage was awry and although Ng'ung'uliko denied it flatly, it was obvious that he had put saliva into his eye.

Why the witchdoctor advised that particular treatment I don't know, but I did know this, the old man's mouth was alive with germs, and after a cataract operation the eye can be very susceptible to this sort of thing.

'Great One,' I said to Ng'ung'uliko, 'why did you disturb your bandage?'

'*Kah*, Bwana,' the old man was surly, '*kah*, I shall go the way that I wish.'

He let loose a tirade of words and got so very excited that I gave him an injection that would put him to sleep before long. But the next day when the bandages were taken off, and the dressing removed, my worst fears were realised – the eye was ruined. Not only had the germs that he had put in done their worst, but the rubbing of the eye had done most serious damage.

'*Keh*,' said the old man, 'I'm in darkness. I'm in darkness. You have deceived me. *Kah*.'

He got out of bed, struggled to his feet, and walked forward, crashing into the wall. He made a wild swipe, knocking over a medicine bottle.

Kefa very quietly took him by the arm. His relations were outside.

'Take me home,' he cried, 'take me away from this place. *Yah*.'

He turned and spat in my direction. We stood silently watching the old man stagger down the path that he should have walked along, seeing. He turned and waved his fist at me, yelling curses at the top of his voice.

'*Hongo*, Bwana,' said Daudi, 'it was he who disobeyed your word. It is he who is saying these things about you.'

'*Kumbe*,' said Kefa, 'is that not always the way? Do not people refuse to go God's way and then when they get into trouble, they blame God when it is their own fault? He has given them a will to choose their way. They choose their way and blame Him and get into trouble.'

Old Ng'wagu was behind me. 'Bwana,' he said, 'when will it be time to work on my eye?'

'Great One,' I said, 'you have heard the trouble we have just had. Do you still wish for me to work upon you?'

'*Heh*, Bwana, I do indeed. Behold, I will follow your words. I will not put *mate*, spit, into my eyes. *Kumbe*, have we not seen today the foolishness of going the wrong way?'

'*Heh*, remember the words of God, "There is a way that seems right to a man, but in the end it leads to death."'

'Truly,' said Daudi, 'and on the way to death, misery and wretchedness.'

'*Kumbe*,' said Ng'wagu, 'I will look on the other side. I will follow your ways, Bwana, that there may be light, and with light, *heh*, I will have joy.'

Next morning, Ng'wagu was still of the same mind.

'Let us just check things,' I said.

Once again I pointed his head into the full glare of the equatorial sun. One eye was clearly beyond hope, but the other…

'What can you see?'

'Bwana, I can see the sun in the sky like a smoky lantern.'

'Nothing more?'

'*Ng'o, ng'o*, Bwana, that and only that.'

'*Yah*, and in five day's time, Great One, there will be a different story.'

16
Light

I shone the torch into Ng'wagu's eyes and turned the lids back. There was not the slightest sign of inflammation anywhere.

'Great One, I think tomorrow at dawn will be the best time to work. But once again, let us go through your routine.

'Look down.' He looked smoothly down.

'Up.' Up the eyes came.

'Your ear.' I touched one side of his face. The eyes moved in that direction.

'Good, and now will you be ready for anything that may happen?'

'Bwana, before you go, talk with God.'

Together we prayed.

'I will give you a little pill,' I said after I got up from my knees.

'Bwana, there will be no need. Behold, I will sleep for I know that *Mulungu*, God Himself, is with me, therefore I have no fear. *Heh*, truly I will sleep well.'

Opening the door of the operating theatre next morning, I was greeted by Daudi.

'Bwana, the old man's eyes look splendid. He slept very well indeed. He is already in the theatre and is lying there very quietly. I have put in some cocaine and I think, Bwana, that there never was a patient more ready than he.'

I went in. '*Mbukwa*, good morning.'

'*Mbukwa*, Bwana. I am in your hands.'

Very carefully I washed his eye out, put more drops in and touched it with a wisp of cotton wool.

'Did you feel anything?'

'*Heh*, Bwana, nothing.'

I put a piece of gauze over his face, and cut a hole in it just large enough for the eye, and put more drops into the eye while I checked over the various instruments with Daudi. He held up the knife that we had previously selected.

'Bwana, we have used it only on Ng'ung'uliko.'

'*Heh*,' I said, 'that will be all right.' Then I turned to the old man. 'Are you ready?'

He nodded.

'Well, before I work we will talk to God.' I nodded to Daudi and he prayed:

'O God, please help the Bwana. May your hand be on his that it may make no mistake or have any tremble in it. May Your hand be upon Ng'wagu that he may hear the instructions of the Bwana and follow them through. Grant that nothing unusual may happen in the operating time, and help in the days of stillness until the bandage is removed.'

Ng'wagu's voice chimed in, 'And oh, Great God, that I may have the light back in my eye.'

I stood at the end of the operating table, Daudi on my right giving me the instruments necessary, and Kefa on the other side to tell the old man what to do.

'Look down, Ng'wagu, at your feet. Keep looking down. You will feel me pressing, but no pain.'

Daudi gave me the eye knife, and the first all-important part of the operation was over in a matter of seconds.

'Good, keep looking down. Now you will feel more pain as though the prick of a thorn came upon your eye. Do not move fast.'

Daudi gave me two delicate instruments and the second stage of the operation was over. The old man continued to look down, but I saw the gauze billowing over his mouth.

'Bwana,' he said in a soft tone, 'Bwana, I want to swallow my spit.'

I looked at Daudi's face. He had a broad grin.

'You may swallow.'

The old man's Adam's apple moved up and down rhythmically, and then he said:

'Bwana, I am ready.'

'This, Great One, is the important stage. Look down, keep very quiet and behold, we will remove it.'

With two instruments carefully I manipulated, and out from the eye smoothly came the cataract. The old man seemed suddenly to be in trouble.

'Bwana,' he said, 'I have cramp, cramp, in my southern leg!'

'*Hongo*,' I said, 'then stretch out your southern heel – stretch it hard and Kefa will rub your leg.'

There was a difficult half-minute. There could have been no worse time for cramp to have taken the old man, but he was comfortable again and the internal structure of the eye was suitably sorted out. Everything was in order. Drops were put in. A gauze pad covered the eye and the bandage was adjusted.

'*Yah*,' said the old man, 'for a moment, Bwana, much light came in, very white light, such as I have not seen for years.'

'Great One, in four days' time more light will come.'

I put between his thumb and finger his cataract.

'There is the thing that blocked. Hold that, and think of it in these days. Think of the blockage of the light.'

'*Heh*, Bwana, I will not forget. I will remember that only you could remove that. I am not forgetful of the cataract of my soul.'

Once again Daudi and I stood at the door of the theatre and watched the old man being carried to the ward.

'Remember, Ng'wagu,' called Daudi, 'for four days lie still, no movement whatsoever, even should the bed bite you.'

The afternoon of the third day the bandage slipped a little. Ng'wagu was agogo when I did my evening round. He beckoned to me:

'Bwana, I saw strong red light when they put on a new bandage! *Yoh*, tomorrow when you take it off completely, then…' His voice trailed off into a dream of what was to be.

It was the late afternoon of the next day when I arrived at the ward. Ng'wagu was tremendously excited. As I scrubbed my hands, he talked:

'*Kah*, Bwana, how I have waited for you. *Heh*…'

'Here I am, Great One, now within five minutes your bandages will be off, but first…' I turned to Daudi. 'Get Kefa to help you. Carry his bed to the veranda. Place it so that he faces the sunset.'

This was done and Daudi ran back to bring out the dressing tray. While Kefa lifted our old patient's head, gently I undid the bandage.

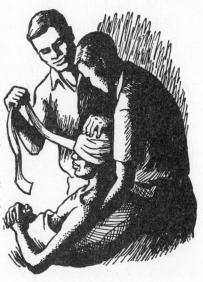

'*Kah*, Bwana,' came Ng'wagu's tense voice, 'it is loose, hope grows…'

The tapes were undone and the cataract bandage came off.

'*Yoh*, it is off, Bwana, and still all is dark.'

I looked across at Daudi and smiled.

'Have patience, Great One, the eye is still covered with cotton wool.'

Very gently I lifted this off with forceps.

'*Yoh*,' came Ng'wagu's voice, hoarse with disappointment, 'you have failed completely. I am still blind.'

Daudi grinned across at me and chuckled.

Ng'wagu abruptly sat up. '*Kah*, you laugh. You, Bwana and your helpers. Your mouths are full of words of light.' He shook his fists at us. '*Yoh*, Berenge failed also. He took my cattle and goats and brought me no light but, *hongo!* He did not laugh at me. *Kah!*...'

'*Pole, pole*, gently, Great One,' I said quietly, 'quench your anger for a small minute.' I looked over my shoulder. 'Daudi, a moist swab, please, his eyelids are only stuck together.'

Using the lightest pressure, I bathed his matted eye lashes. They slowly came apart and the eyes opened.

Anger and disappointment vanished in a split second. An amazed smile came over the old man's face as his eye slowly opened.

'*Hongo*, Bwana, there *is* light. I can see. I – can – see!'

We stood back against the wall and in the dim light Daudi said, 'Great One, tell me, who can you see?'

'*Kah*,' said the old man peering. '*Yah*,' he said, 'I can see the Bwana. Is not his shirt white, and his face above it? And next to him, it is one with a blue shirt. Behold, I can see. Let me look through the window that I may see the countryside, the cattle, the baobab trees, my country.'

'Great One,' I said coming forward with the eye-dropper, 'tomorrow you shall see that. Tonight, rest in the knowledge that light has come back to your eyes.'

The old man held up a wisp of cotton wool, in it the eye lens.

'Bwana, this was the thing that stopped me from seeing. That little thing blocked the light, but now it has gone, light has come. *Kumbe*, Bwana, it has come to me: how well I can understand now what sin is! *Kah*, did you not say that it blocked the light of God from coming in? It was the barrier, the blockage. *Kah*, I understand it.'

'Truly He is the Light of the World.'

Further down the ward I could see Tadayo looking at me. 'Bwana, remember the day *nje*, the scorpion, bit me?'

I nodded.

'You spoke of a warning against a secret sin. *Kumbe!* This was a cataract in my soul's eye, but *heeh!* He has removed it. My heart is full, Bwana. May I sing?' I nodded. He burst into song: 'I will not stop singing.' Everybody joined in the chorus and by the time they had finished singing, I had the bandage back on the old man's eye. He was settling back comfortably in bed and Kefa was rubbing his back with methylated spirits.

A week passed and Ng'wagu was walking about the hospital now with a crudely made cardboard eye-shield keeping the glare out of his newly repaired eye, as he liked to call it. He walked around giving people demonstrations of what he could do. I had seen him walk almost into a thornbush, and then stop and laugh, and say:

'*Heeh*, see, I no longer walk into it?'

He would walk to the very edge of a hole and then on the brink he would cry:

'*Yah*, there was a time not long ago when I would have fallen in, but now, *heh*, I can see.'

In the evening he would walk very near to the camp fire and stop just short of the living coals.

'*Heh*, behold, my feet do not get burnt. Can I not see?'

Night after night I had heard him tell of what it meant for him to be able to see.

Then he was ready to go home. He took my hand in both of his and shook it.

'Bwana,' he said, 'you have given me great joy. Behold, I can return along the safari to my home, seeing the way, and Bwana, as I walk that road I will think of the path that I travel to God. I walk in the light now and I will obey Him and His way. The words shall be read to me from His Book. *Kah*, Bwana, I would never have understood these things properly but for your little knife and the operation.'

It was the next morning at sunrise that he set out. I watched the old man walk off into the reddening east. In two senses a new day was dawning for him.

The rains came and the whole countryside was busy planting millet, planting maize, planting peanuts. The countryside rang with the rhythm of the hoe and the songs of the people as they put in their seed.

Daudi was beside me.

'Bwana,' he said, 'behold, when the crops have grown and the corn is safely gathered in, then we will see more people at the hospital, and Bwana, perhaps then Ng'wagu will visit us again. I have heard word today that he is working for the first time in ten years, with shoes of his village, and that his hoe moves as it has never moved before. *Yah*, Bwana, they say he is full of new songs.'

17
Walking in the Light

The last thunderstorm of the wet season had deluged Central Tanganyika. Everything was green and then in two weeks the burning heat of the sun turned the whole countryside from green to brown. The crops ripened and in every village the harvest songs were sung.

The dry cornstalks were raked together. Fires sprang up in the darkness all over the place as they were burnt off, and again the songs of the tribes came musically over the plains.

I had been late in the hospital doing eye dressings, when suddenly a different sound came on the night air.

'*Hongo,*' said Kefa, 'it sounds like the lorry of Sulimani.'

A long toot on the horn underlined this and a few minutes later the lorry drew up outside the hospital.

'Good evening, sir,' said Sulimani, 'I was passing through Dodoma and I met two friends of yours and I brought them here. They would have suffered in the journey, so I invited them to travel in the back of my lorry.'

An old man with cowhide sandals had scrambled to the ground and was helping down another old man who obviously was blind. I went across to the greet them. The first old man came across to me.

'Bwana,' he said, 'it is I, Ng'wagu. I have returned with one from my village who would also have you work on him. Bwana, I have joy. My eye works well. *Heh*, I have light. Have I not heard the word, "If we walk in the light as Jesus is in the light, we have fellowship one with the other"? Bwana, I learnt that here first, and *kah*, I have found it true these days.'

I gripped him by the hand.

'My friend, it is joy to see you.'

We led the new patient into the ward and he was put to bed awaiting the usual preparation.

Ng'wagu said, 'I will sleep, Bwana, on the floor beside him. He has fears, but I will help him. I will train him as Kefa trained me. Behold, Bwana, in this way I will help him into the light. *Kumbe*, Bwana, he too has walked into the fire and fallen down holes as I have. Life to him is a burden. He cannot work in his garden or help with the harvest. He just sits in the darkness, Bwana, and I have brought him to you for healing. *Kumbe*, have I not told him the stories that I learnt about Jesus here? He has felt the lens that you took from my eyes. I have taken him to hear the words

154

of God at the C.M.S. Village School, and have we not come a four-day journey to seek your help?'

'You shall both be helped,' I said. 'You, Ng'wagu, we will teach new songs, that your heart may be full of gladness, and you...'

'Bwana,' said the old man, 'Cibofu is my name. I am the blind one.'

'You, we will help in the way of the hospital.'

'*Assante*, thank you,' said both the old men together. It was pathetic to see the eagerness of Ng'wagu to take care of his friend. He carefully went through all the routine of preparation for operation. When the great day arrived, he asked rather diffidently if he might come to the theatre. I readily agreed.

He was given a cap and mask and sat on a stool in the corner, and before I started, as usual we prayed.

Ng'wagu added his postscript to the prayer, 'And please God let him see once again as I see now.'

The operation went very smoothly.

'*Yoh*, Bwana,' smiled Daudi as we fixed the bandages in position, 'Kefa will need to watch his step. Ng'wagu is certainly a good one to train those who require their darkness to be removed.'

'*Hongo*,' said the patient as we lifted him on to the stretcher, 'truly, he is a helpful one.'

'*Ngheeh*,' agreed Daudi. 'Now you follow his words for the next four days and do not follow the ways of Ng'ung'uliko, the grumbler, who removed his bandage and put spit into his eye and ruined the Bwana's work.'

Clearly on the still, hot air came a strident voice:

'*Kah!* The Bwana did me no good. I, Ng'ung'uliko, say his medicines are of small strength.'

Kefa's indignant tones broke in. 'You are blind still, because you did not obey the words of the *fundi*, the expert. The fault is not his but yours. *Yoh!* Sow spit in your eye and you harvest blindness; sow pumpkins in your garden and you get pumpkins; sow sin in you life and you get death, with pain, disappointment and misery on the way.

'The Bible says, "Do not be deceived: God cannot be mocked. A man reaps what he sows." You planted, now reap your harvest, bitter though it is, and don't grumble.'

Daudi and I turned away and went to the ward where our patient was just being put to bed.

'*Kumbe*, Bwana, is not Ng'ung'uliko like the man who heard God's word and did not obey it? And is not Ng'wagu like the man who heard and obeyed? One built solidly, the other built to fall.'

In the ward Ng'wagu was sitting beside his friend who was lying in bed.

'Keep quiet,' he said. 'Lie very still. Should you want a drink, just tell me. If you have places that itch, I will scratch them for you. Whatever you do, do not move your hands to your face. I will be here to help you.'

How effectively he helped can be judged by the fact that just over a week later, I saw two old men walk through the door of the Children's Ward, and come to a stop before the picture of "The Light of the World."

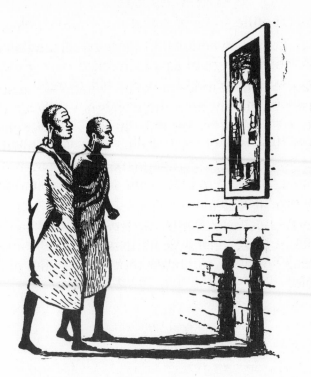

'That is Jesus,' said Ng'wagu. 'He is outside the door of your heart. He says, *"Hodi?* May I come in?"* And when you reply *"Karibu,"* He comes in and in comes light, as light came into your eye when the Bwana removed the block.'

'*Hongo*,' said Cibofu. 'Truly, I will say *"Karibu"* to Him that He may do to my life what He has done to yours. *Heh*, He has worked strongly there.'

I came in and stood beside them.

'Bwana,' said Ng'wagu, 'my friend understands now. Truly your little knife makes it very easy for him, too.'

'*Heh*, Cibofu?'

'*Mbeka*, truly, Bwana, and I have asked the Son of God to work in my life as you worked on my eyes. *Kumbe*, Bwana, we are both too old to read God's Book but our grandchildren are going to the C.M.S. School. They will read to us so that we may know how to follow Him, so that we may obey Him as we obeyed you.'

'*Kumbe*, Bwana,' old Ng'wagu stood very straight, 'surely we, the people of Africa, have been blind in our hearts for many, many years. *Kah*, but you have brought to many, many of us here the Light. Truly, Bwana, your little knife works very strongly. It is sharper in its preaching than many tongues.'

THE JUNGLE DOCTOR SERIES

CHRISTIAN FOCUS PUBLICATIONS

Christian Focus   Christian Heritage   CF4K   Mentor

Christian Focus Publications publishes books for adults and children under its four main imprints: Christian Focus, CF4K, Mentor and Christian Heritage. Our books reflect our conviction that God's Word is reliable and Jesus is the way to know him, and live for ever with him.

Our children's publication list includes a Sunday School curriculum that covers pre-school to early teens, and puzzle and activity books. We also publish personal and family devotional titles, biographies and inspirational stories that children will love.

If you are looking for quality Bible teaching for children then we have an excellent range of Bible stories and age-specific theological books.

From pre-school board books to teenage apologetics, we have it covered!

Find us at our web page:
www.christianfocus.com

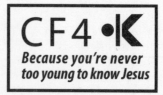

CF4 •K
Because you're never too young to know Jesus